LOUISE GRAHAM PhD

CAN I HAVE CHIPS?

FILL UP   LOSE WEIGHT   FEEL GREAT

Matador
9 Priory Business Park
Kibworth Beauchamp
Leicestershire LE8 0RX, UK
Tel: (+44) 116 279 2299
Fax: (+44) 116 279 2277
Email: books@troubador.co.uk
Web: www.troubador.co.uk/matador

ISBN 978 1783062 423

British Library Cataloguing in Publication Data.
A catalogue record for this book is available from the British Library.

Typeset by Troubador Publishing Ltd
Printed and bound in the UK by TJ International, Padstow, Cornwall

Matador is an imprint of Troubador Publishing Ltd

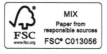

For Jack

ABOUT THE AUTHOR

Louise Graham was educated at London University. Her first degree was in physiology. She then studied at the Institute of Obstetrics and Gynaecology and obtained a PhD in clinical pharmacology. She was awarded a post doctoral fellowship at the Royal Postgraduate Medical School, Hammersmith Hospital and has contributed to papers on neonatal jaundice published by the *British Medical Journal*, the *Lancet* and the *Journal of Clinical Pharmacology*. She has written two books – one on nutrition.

After years of yo-yo dieting, Louise used her research skills to develop a realistic and sustainable weight loss plan. Following extensive trials, she refined her method on her long suffering husband and three sons who were never sure what they would be eating for dinner.

Louise is on a mission to show overweight people, whatever their background or level of income, how easy it is to lose weight and more importantly keep it off.

She currently works as a holistic therapist in London.

For more information, visit www.canihavechips.co.uk.

Also by Louise Graham

A Good Start (Penguin Books)
George's First Year (Peter Halban)

A little of what you fancy does you good
Proverb

ACKNOWLEDGEMENTS

I would like to acknowledge with gratitude my husband Richard for his constructive criticism and encouragement.

Thanks are due to Rosemary Friedman and Susan Grossman for help with the manuscript. Lastly to Shaun Aspinall and his team of willing guinea pigs who road tested the diet in its early stages and provided valuable feedback.

CONTENTS

PREFACE

The relationship we have with food is intriguing as much as it is complex. We are pulled by two opposing forces: the pressure to have a perfect body and the desire to eat pizza and ice cream. Guess which one inevitably wins! We follow the latest faddy diet and breathe a sigh of relief as we squeeze back into that too tight skirt or pair of trousers. We lap up the compliments of friends or colleagues and everything in the garden is rosy – at least for a while. But behaviours are not easily changed, hunger soon gets the better of us and the pounds pile back on.

Obesity research has yet to come up with a definitive answer as to why we eat too much, or even a consensus as to what makes us fat. While the experts seek to incriminate sugar, then fat, then sugar again, we gain more weight. If we want to know how to be slim, we must turn to the naturally slim for the answers. Whilst some have a genetic predisposition, many do not. What are their eating habits? What do they choose to eat? Emulate them and surely permanent weight reduction must follow. But how, when we know that behaviour is notoriously hard to modify and constant dieting makes us progressively fatter?

Tell us to hunt down juniper berries, lemon grass or venison burgers, and before long we are back to our old eating patterns. But show us a healthy and filling diet that offsets the increase in appetite and craving for carbohydrates triggered by calorie restriction, and dieting becomes a whole new ball game.

We have lost the wood for the trees. Dieting for dieting's sake is no longer enough. If we wish to be shadows of our former selves, it is time to eat less and eat better. Not rocket science – but quite a challenge.

INTRODUCTION

Do you yearn to be able to wear all the clothes in your wardrobe, and gaze at your skinny friends with envy wondering how they manage it? Welcome to the club. Yet the reason is clear, they eat less, just watch them at mealtimes or look into their shopping trolleys – no matter how much you are deluding yourself to the contrary.

Give your full attention to the main reason why you never get any slimmer – you find it too challenging. Don't be too hard on yourself though; the idea that eating little but meat, obsessively counting calories or semi fasting two days a week can result in permanent weight loss is laughable. Faddy short term diets lead to rebound weight gain, as your body thinks that it is starving and releases hormones that stimulate the appetite. Yet without a reduction in the energy content of your diet you will not lose any weight. But first we need to understand why we are eating too much.

Forty years ago overeating was unusual, particularly amongst children and young adults, and this gives us a clue as to the most likely dietary causes. The obesity time bomb coincides with the increased consumption of foods containing added sugar and added fat, larger portions and eating away from home. Naturally slim people snack less, and eat more wholegrains, fish, poultry, fruits and vegetables. When they dine out, they frequent full service restaurants rather than fast food outlets. Or they eat little – a strategy followed through necessity by millions of people in parts of the world where there is not enough to eat.

Firstly let's quash a common misconception that to lose weight you must avoid carbohydrates. Not true – just the ones you love – confectionary, cakes, biscuits, pies, pizzas and pastries. These fat laden offerings are both energy rich and highly palatable, making it difficult to only eat a little. Neither do you have to join the gym in order to lose weight. People who love to do sport are generally slim and have loads of energy to burn. They are not slim because they exercise.

Obesity is a metabolic disorder resulting in low energy levels, and being instructed to work out or pound the pavements can leave you more exhausted and heading straight for your favourite sugary fix. Of course, being active raises your metabolic rate and improves fitness and muscle tone, but modest exercise makes much less difference to your weight than reducing your energy intake.

No need then for yo-yo dieting and a fat and thin wardrobe. Ditch the fast foods, sugary drinks and snacks, and eat three filling meals a day. But you are rarely at home, have little inclination to cook and the only piece of kitchen equipment you possess is a microwave. No excuse – you can eat out and still lose weight, although you save money and slim down faster if you can cook simple dishes.

Okay, so you understand the principle: ditch those choc chip muffins and savoury snacks, and a slender body is yours. But you love eating, and snacking is one of your favourite activities – and I don't mean on an apple or carrot. Find yourself unable to turn away from the tasty, fatty foods you crave? Being less powerful than a Krispy Kreme doughnut is nothing to be proud of.

In the dieting game sustainable weight loss is the Holy Grail, not how quickly you shed those excess pounds.

YES, YOU CAN HAVE CHIPS!

Bob's Story

Bob the builder is a big man. In his van he keeps a stash of snacks to boost his energy levels. Desperate to lose weight so that he can kick a football around with his son without becoming puffed out, he is excited about the prospect of dieting because he knows he can still enjoy his favourite food – chips.

Including a food Bob likes makes it easier for him to stick to the diet. Although they are deep fried, even the greasiest chips are lower in energy per gram than pastry or biscuits because of their water content. They fill him up and one small portion a day does not prevent weight loss. On days he doesn't have chips; Bob is permitted one square of plain dark chocolate after lunch and dinner, but not milk chocolate which is high in added sugar and low in healthy cocoa.

Weighing in at 19 stone 8 lbs, he has a body mass index of thirty-eight, putting him firmly in the obese range. Like many people on low income he subsists on cheap calories, which leaves him enough money at the end of the week to go to the pub with his mates.

He hasn't eaten meat and two veg since he was at primary school, and he thinks that if he wants to lose weight he will be expected to give up his beloved cooked breakfast and eat muesli instead. Regular cups of tea with sugar are a lifelong habit. As is finishing everything on his plate, because that was what his mother had insisted upon.

The more he worries about his size and the discomfort it causes him, the less he is able to do anything about it. He doesn't like his job and sometimes suffers from depression. He wants to be a foreman but he isn't good with people. The worse his mood, the more he eats, as it makes him feel better, at least temporarily.

Bob's Typical Daily Food Intake

Weekday:

- Breakfast – porridge or Weetabix, two cups of tea with two sugars
- Mid morning – builders' fry up, one cup of tea with two sugars, one soft drink
- Lunch – cooked meal, one cup of tea with two sugars, one soft drink
- Afternoon snacks – crisps, confectionary, one soft drink
- Evening meal – large main course with pudding, one soft drink

- After dinner – crisps, chocolate, strawberry trifle, cake
- Fruit – three bananas a day
- He visits the pub three or four nights a week and drinks up to ten pints of beer per visit.

Weekend:

- Takeaways – fish and chips, Chinese or McDonalds
- Sunday roast
- Tea with two sugars, soft drinks and snacks
- Fruit – three bananas a day

Bob understands that to lose weight successfully he needs to lower his energy intake by cutting down on foods containing added sugar and added fat, and curb his appetite by upping his intake of protein. He is encouraged to deal more effectively with life's ups and downs, rather than using food as an emotional crutch.

He starts eating three meals a day, each consisting of a serving of protein, one standard mug (250ml) of starchy food and unlimited vegetables and fresh fruit. He avoids snacks and soft drinks, stops adding sugar to his tea and cuts his alcohol consumption to one drink a day. He begins to lose weight immediately and in just five weeks is 23lbs lighter. He starts the maintenance plan and three months later he has not regained the lost weight. No longer craving an unlimited supply of sugary, fatty food, he is ready to start another round of weight loss.

Amanda's Story

Amanda – a mother – has been overweight for as long as she can remember. Yo-yo dieting is her style. She often tries calorie counting, but claims that no matter how few calories she eats, she doesn't get any thinner. Attempts at cutting out carbohydrates are effective but give her a headache, make her grumpy and tired, and her efforts never last more than a week.

Weighing in at 13 stone 2lbs, her body mass index is twenty-eight, putting her in the overweight range.

She enjoys cooking, but her diet is limited and small portions are an alien concept.

Like many stay at home mothers she indulges in sugary and fatty treats to help her cope with the daily stresses of looking after her family. She thinks potatoes are fattening and fills up on sliced white toast with honey, as she considers honey to be good for her. Having mid morning elevenses with chocolate biscuits is a ritual, and rarely an afternoon goes by without a cream tea. She raids the fridge at night when woken by a crying child.

Her wardrobe is full of clothes that she hopes to get back into one day and she is reluctant to have a clear out. She is reminded about her weight each day when she gets dressed and tries to find something to wear.

Being at home all day with the children makes Amanda feel unfulfilled. A feeling she tries to stifle by filling herself with food.

Amanda's Typical Daily Food Intake

- Breakfast – toast and jam, or sugary cereal and milk
- Elevenses – chocolate biscuits and milky coffee
- Lunch – cheese, soup or hummus with several slices of mass produced bread, fruit
- Afternoon tea – scones with cream and jam
- Dinner – meat, potatoes and vegetables or takeaway curry followed by chocolate mousse or large helping of ice cream. Two large glasses of wine
- After dinner – chocolate and cake

Amanda realises that she needs to stop snacking and value the important role she plays as a mother. Feeling better about herself makes her less inclined to fill herself up with rubbish.

Amanda prepares to make the transition to three meals a day and no snacks, choosing to take it one step at a time. She cuts back her wine consumption to one glass a day and curbs her night time eating habit. Four weeks later she is 14lbs lighter. After six months she has lost two stone. She proceeds to the maintenance plan. A year later she has not regained the lost weight and can even get into some of the clothes she 'grew' out of. Her new way of eating has become a way of life that she enjoys and does not intend to give up.

Peter's Story

A fat baby, Peter grew into a fat child, a fat teenager and then a fat young man. To get him through his working day as a labourer on a building site he relies on energy drinks, cigarettes and coffee. His partner does all the cooking and he eats everything that is put in front of him. He often visits his mother who loves nothing better than spoiling him with the cakes and biscuits that featured so heavily during his childhood.

His favourite leisure activity is drinking at his local pub. He would like to take up running but is too embarrassed about his size. He weighs 16 stone 8lbs and has a body mass index of thirty-two, putting him in the obese range.

He never diets because he doesn't know how to, and obesity runs in his family. Now he is a daddy, he doesn't want his baby son having to cope with the taunts of 'fatty' he received from the other children at school. He is keen to set him a good example and is eager to start the diet.

Peter's Typical Daily Food Intake

- Breakfast – none
- Lunch – none
- Drinks – water, two energy drinks or cola, three cups of coffee with one sugar
- Tea – crackers, cheese, crisps, biscuits
- Dinner – meat and two vegetables (home cooked) with a lot of white bread, two cans of lager

- After dinner – chocolate bar
- He visits the pub three times a week, drinking fourteen cans of lager per week.

Peter knows that to lose weight successfully he needs to learn about nutrition. He finds the dietary information described in CAN I HAVE CHIPS? easy to understand.

He gives up sugar, soft drinks and between meal snacks, and eats three protein rich meals a day. Before leaving home in the morning he has porridge and a handful of almonds. He makes a packed lunch of pasta, cheese and raw vegetables to take to work. For dinner he cooks meat, potatoes and vegetables, or sausage, egg and chips followed by fresh fruit. He cuts his pub visits to once a week.

His energy levels soar as his weight begins to drop. After five weeks he has lost 13lbs. After eight months he is two stone lighter and is on the maintenance plan.

Peter is happy with his new way of eating and feels confident in the knowledge that he now has the skills to lose more weight when he is ready. He makes sure that his little boy is eating healthy home cooked meals which include fruit and vegetables, so that history does not repeat itself.

PART ONE

Get Motivated

2

THE ART OF EATING LESS

Have you lost weight only to put it straight back on again? You are not alone – less than 5% of slimmers manage to keep weight off for longer than five years, but there are good reasons for this. You need a combination of both mental and physical changes to succeed at long term weight loss.

Dieting makes you hungry because your body thinks that it is starving and releases ghrelin, a hormone that increases your appetite. Ghrelin levels do not return to normal until you have maintained your new weight for at least six months, making rebound weight gain an inevitable consequence of faddy, short term diets. Yo-yo diet and you end up a little fatter each time. But change your behaviour and follow a satisfying and sustainable eating plan that compensates for this natural increase in appetite and you need never go on another diet!

Understanding why you are overweight is the first step to having the body you desire. Although eating processed foods containing added sugar and fat predispose you to obesity they are not the sole cause of your predicament. If that were true there would not be so many skinny fast food junkies – most of them active young men!

As portion sizes grow and plates groan with food, it is inevitable that you expand as well. Breakfast at the Ritz, dine at the Dorchester or frequent your local burger bar and chippie, it makes no difference; if you want to weigh less, you must cut back on calories whatever their source, or start training for the marathon. This skill is fundamental to successful dieting, and without it slimming down can only be a pipe dream.

Cut back? Not a problem – you've been cutting since you first grasped those blunt, plastic scissors at play school, but like a surgeon you need to know where to focus your incision for maximum effect. Is it better to cut out a protein rich lamb chop or a carbohydrate rich jam sandwich? Protein and carbohydrate contain the same number of calories, but we now know that calories do not tell the full story, because it requires more energy to absorb and digest protein, effectively making it less fattening.

However, this does not mean that carbohydrates make you fat – only eating too much can do that. Just look at the rice eating populations of Southeast Asia with their low levels of obesity. It is the high energy western diet with its reliance on fast foods that is the culprit.

But lamb chops are fatty – surely fat has to be fattening? With more than twice the energy of protein and carbohydrate and easily assimilated at almost no energy cost, it makes sense to discard the visible fat from meat.

Whenever faced with food, perform some judicious cutting. If snacks are your vice – give them up, it is unlikely that you compensate by eating less at your next meal. Cut out takeaways and burn off that spare tyre by wielding a saucepan, a wooden spoon and a sharp knife – it is cheaper than going to the gym. Wean yourself off sugary soft drinks – liquid sugar does not fill you up. Become a water drinker (that's the stuff that comes free out of the tap). But fruit juice is healthy isn't it? True it contains nutrients, but it has the same amount of sugar (from the fruit) as fizzy drinks. Try eating an apple or orange instead – that's one piece of fruit after a meal not the three or four (or even more) in your glass of juice.

Take sugar in your tea? Now is the time to gradually cut down and then stop completely. It may taste unpleasant to begin with, but after a couple of weeks you won't miss it. Eat a protein rich main course and pass on the pudding. Say no to second helpings and stop eating by 9pm or even earlier – this allows your body ten to twelve hours to burn stored energy without it being replenished. Recent scientific studies suggest that late night eating is worse, in terms of weight gain, than eating during normal daylight hours. Cut down on alcohol, it stimulates appetite and promotes fat build up. Limit yourself to one alcoholic drink daily – the type is less important than the quantity.

Curtail your eating out habit, especially at fast food outlets. Owing to the quantity of flavoursome additives in their calorific offerings overconsumption is easy, particularly if you wash your meal down with an oversized soft drink. Calorie counting is arduous and of little help when it comes to losing weight and keeping it off which requires a permanent change in eating habits. It does however come in useful if you just happen to find yourself in a fast food chain. Ask for nutritional information, do your best not to exceed 600kcals per meal, and don't make a habit of it.

Surprised by how little you need to eat in order to trigger weight loss? As you approach middle age, your metabolism slows down due to muscle loss and inactivity, making slimming more of a challenge – so start pumping iron to build up those muscles. Having difficulty eating less? Switch to a less processed diet; you can fill up and still lose weight.

Key Points:

- **Cut portion size**
- **Cut out between meal snacks**
- **Cut out takeaways**
- **Cut out fruit juice and sweetened soft drinks**
- **Cut out sugar in tea and coffee**
- **Cut back on eating out**
- **Cut back on alcohol**
- **Cut night time eating**

3

THE ART OF EATING BETTER

Finding it tedious surviving on reduced rations? Let this useful skill come to the rescue: the art of swapping yummy processed foods for filling and satisfying real foods. Dump the ready meals and switch to a virtuous diet of proteins supplemented with a moderate amount of carbohydrates – grains, pulses, pasta, potatoes, fruits and vegetables (do I hear a yawn?).

No need to fear carbohydrates, they provide you with the energy you need to function and they help to ease the carbohydrate cravings triggered by calorie restriction. Some are high in fibre which makes you feel full and some contain a type of starch (resistant starch) that resists digestion. This means you can eat more of these and weigh less. Pulses, firm bananas and wholegrains are good sources, and so are cold pasta, cold potatoes and deep fried potato products such as hash browns, croquettes and chips. Crisps are high in added fat and low in resistant starch, and are best avoided.

Want to lose weight but not prepared to give up your favourite foods? You may as well resign yourself to eating minute portions of your usual processed diet. Let swapping be your lifeline if you hope to step off the diet treadmill. Call on it every time you eat out, go food shopping or prepare a meal. If you always head straight to the fridge for a sugary dessert after your takeaway, this skill will help. Together with your cutting skill, swapping allows you to make that long overdue move out of your oversized rut.

Snacks and soft drinks are amongst the worst culprits when it comes to weight gain, because they are usually consumed in addition to meals rather than as replacements. You have a stressful morning getting the kids off to school – you eat some left over birthday cake, well it would be a crime to throw it away. The weather is great but your holiday is long way off – that tub of ice cream lurking at the back of the freezer is too tempting to resist. Your boss has made you redundant – out comes the choc chip muffin and smoothie. Don't be conned into thinking that if your snack comes from a health food store, it must be okay. It probably isn't.

You choose food to cheer yourself up, whereas your thinner friends turn to cigarettes, coffee, recreational drugs, compulsive shopping, non-stop TV, excessive exercise or promiscuity. Annoyingly, the results of your addiction are a little more noticeable.

Swap your snacks for filling meals low in added sugar and added fat. You get more than enough sugar in fruits, and plenty of fat in natural foods like meat, fish, dairy and nuts. Eating sufficient at mealtimes stops you feeling peckish. Of course you may snack out of boredom rather than because you are hungry; if that is the case then a distraction is the only solution.

Snacking might not be your scene, but you are not averse

to buying a croissant and your favourite sweetened coffee fix on the way to the office, scoffing a cheeseburger and milkshake for lunch, or picking up a pizza, garlic bread, chicken nuggets and bottle of coke on the way home. Looking for a sure way to gain weight – then eating fast foods is the answer.

Get into the habit of eating breakfast at home – even if it is only a banana, some natural yoghurt and few nuts. If you must buy coffee on the way to work, don't add sugar and ditch the cupcake. Dust off the Tupperware and make a packed lunch – no, you can't swap your apple for a chocolate bar with your colleague. In the evening, dine on sausage, mash and peas, or expensive steak with a quinoa salad; it makes little difference to your rate of weight loss. The fact that you are eating a protein rich, home cooked meal of real food is what counts.

Need to eat out during the day? Then prepare to be discerning. Coffee shops and supermarkets offer a variety of healthy ready to eat foods such as prepared salads or low fat wraps. Fancy something more exotic? Traditional fish sushi is a good compromise, low in added fat and containing a reasonable amount of protein, just don't add mayonnaise. In your staff cafeteria pick cold cuts, meat, fish or eggs, supplemented with potatoes, vegetables, pasta, baked beans or bean salad, followed by fresh fruit. Or have a bowl of soup, some bread and natural yoghurt.

Restaurant food is usually superior in quality to fast food outlets and a lot pricier, so you could be excused for thinking it might help you lose weight. However portions are often generous or swimming in oil (olive of course), and the bread basket and dessert menu are often too delicious to resist.

Occasional visits only please, and don't be surprised if you find yourself heavier the next morning.

Hone your food shopping skills. If it is not in your basket at the checkout, it won't end up in your mouth. Keen on sugary breakfast cereals, pies, biscuits, soft drinks and desserts, or are you partial to designer granola, croissants and posh chocolates? They may cost more, but are just as deadly to the waistline.

Saving precious cooking time is a boon; however many convenience foods and ready meals (glorified leftovers) and almost all prepared desserts must be off limits because they are high in added sugar, fat or both. Whatever your budget; rule number one is to purchase fresh or minimally processed foods. This restricts you to a very small proportion of what is on sale in your local supermarket and requires steely determination. Just keep repeating the mantra 'but you're worth it', shop without your partner or children, buy online, or frequent your local farmers' market.

Processed foods tend to be cheaper than fresh foods. Often found on special offer, their appeal is understandable particularly if you are buying one and getting one free. But where there's a will there's a way, and it is possible to spend no more on fresh foods than you would on ready meals. To mitigate serious damage to your wallet, look out for late night bargains and reduced price food approaching its sell-by-date. Store perishables correctly and stop throwing away fruit and vegetables when they look a bit tired. Stew fruit and make soup with the vegetables. Given that you are now shunning the sweets and chocolates at the checkout, you may even find that your shopping bill goes down.

Fruit and vegetables are an essential part of successful weight loss because they are fat free and mostly water. Yes, that's those green, red and yellow things that you tend to ignore in your rush to uncover the delights of the confectionary aisle. Fruit fulfils your desire for sweetness – given that you are aiming to give up sugary foods; and vegetables are bulky. Aim for two vegetables at lunch and dinner and a piece of fruit for dessert. No need for trendy veggies and hot housed tomatoes; your stomach won't be able to tell the difference.

Eat what's in season and home grown, even if you are sick of the sight of carrots and cabbage. It usually tastes better and has a lower carbon footprint. If the thought of preparing greens is too much of a chore and you have plenty of spare cash, buy ready prepared veggies. All you have to do is pop them in the microwave. Frozen fruits and vegetables are labour saving and are often more nutritious than fresh.

On shopping expeditions, avert your gaze from the buttery croissants, soft white bread, unctuous scones and fruity tea cakes, and hunt out the hearty pumpernickel, chewy sourdough, earnest stoneground or wholegrain bread. You will get used to them, I promise. These breads are rich in fibre and resistant starch which fill you up and help you lose weight. If white or brown is all that your local shop offers, let it stale for a day or two before consumption, which makes it less fattening – if you can wait that long for your toast.

Swap your favourite jam and honey for nut butters. High in protein, consuming nuts regularly helps you control your weight, and you are less likely to want elevenses. Keen on cereals? Trade in your sugary cereals and greasy granolas for muesli, porridge or low sugar, high fibre cereals. Or eat a cooked breakfast, but skip the fried bread or replace it with a slice of brown toast.

Bid farewell to those appetising pasties, cheese burgers or fried chicken – popular choices for a work day lunch, and say hello to mixed bean salad and cold meat, smoked fish with grainy bread, or hearty soup and a banana. Stop ogling that lemon tart, eclair or chocolate pudding, and swap them for a piece of cheese, or that old standby – natural yoghurt. Can't resist temptation? Then you can forget about losing weight – that is unless you plan on starving the rest of the day (or possibly week).

Cook your own meals – and take control of the ingredients. The weather is freezing and you need warming up with a slug of carbohydrate. Swap fatty pastry based dishes for a standard serving of meat, fish, tofu, Quorn, cheese, eggs or pulses accompanied by one standard mug (250ml) of fat free cooked potatoes, pasta, rice, quinoa, barley, couscous or millet. Add your favourite vegetables and a low fat sauce such as black bean, tomato, or mango. In hot weather, eat your carbohydrates cold, preferably after they have been stored in the fridge for twenty-four hours. This increases the amount of resistant starch they contain. Wanting a sweet dessert is normal; try fresh or stewed fruit instead.

Reclaiming a slimmer body requires a new way of eating. It doesn't happen overnight. Whenever tempted by the processed foods you crave, swap them for real foods. Having problems trading your chocolate bar for a banana? Some skilful planning may be more to your liking.

Key Points:

- Replace processed foods with real foods
- Replace snacks with breakfast, lunch and dinner
- Replace sugary desserts with fruit
- Replace jam and honey with nut and seed butters
- Replace eating out with home cooked meals

4

THE ART OF CREATING STRATEGIES

As if on autopilot your hand hovers over your crisps, shifting from packet to mouth without pause. Your knife and fork dance in perpetual motion, stopping only when your plate is wiped clean. A bag of sweets jumps seamlessly into your basket at the checkout. You open your kitchen cupboard and a packet of chocolate biscuits falls out. Want to be slimmer? Create some cunning strategies.

Stand on the scales regularly – a quick reminder of any indiscretion. Stop buying fizzy drinks, biscuits and little treats; out of sight is out of mind. When faced with junk foods, mutter 'I can resist temptation' until the urge begins to dissipate. The stresses of daily life coupled with a plentiful supply of food make this a strategy that you ignore at your peril.

Eat with a knife and fork and put them down between mouthfuls. Pay attention to what passes your lips. Distractions like watching TV or reading when eating lead to an increase in the number of calories consumed at that meal and later on in the day.

Off to do your weekly shop? Prepare a shopping list and

stick to it. Cook from scratch and you are bound to think twice about how much fat, sugar and salt you are eating. But beware; homemade meals can put the brakes on weight loss – particularly if you are seduced by sexy TV chefs who do not hold back on their mouth watering creations.

Learn the basics of nutrition – the knowledge that not all foods are created equal underpins successful slimming. Fat is high in calories, containing more than twice the energy of protein and carbohydrate, and minimal energy is required for assimilation. Protein is the hardest for your body to process and is more filling than carbohydrate or fat making it a very effective weight loss tool. So don't just cook your favourite dish assuming that it will help you shed the pounds – it may not. But be mindful of what you are going to cook and it just might.

For simple day to day cooking, build a repertoire of soups, salads, roasts, grills and stews low in added fat. Added fat includes oil, margarine, butter, cream, salad dressing and even low fat spreads which are still fats. Fat contributes to the energy content and palatability of food. Limit fat rich desserts to special occasions or when you reach your weight loss goal and are maintaining your weight.

Eating out? Find a venue that serves real food. Decide in advance not to have those tempting sweets or chocolates that are served with coffee. Study the menu online before going out. Once at the restaurant you risk getting side tracked after a drink or two, and ordering dishes high in added fat. The cheaper the restaurant the larger the portions, so compensate by eating abstemiously earlier in the day. Persuade yourself that your enforced self denial means that you can relax and enjoy your meal out. Rumbling stomach? Stay at your desk, read a book, do the ironing or have a cup of tea. Alternatively, ask for a doggie bag.

Off on holiday – that can only mean loads of food and alcohol. Don't expect to snack all day and drink unlimited cocktails without consequences. Relax, but don't take your eye of the ball or should I say stomach. There is little more soul destroying than coming home from holiday half a stone heavier. Lessen the risk of undoing all your good work by choosing self catering and actually using the kitchen.

Booked full board? Then be afraid, very afraid, and approach the dining room with utmost caution. Practise damage limitation by avoiding foods that are deep fried, involve pastry or contain a lot of added sugar and fat. Favour grilled fish or meat, eggs, bread, potatoes, rice, pasta, pulses, cheese and vegetables. Salad is healthy, as long as you ask for dressing to be served separately and only take a little. For dessert: ice cream (one scoop), sorbet, mousse or fresh fruit are your best options.

Dive straight in to your meals without a moment's pause and you have little hope of changing your habitual response. Every time you are faced with food, ask yourself:

- Is it real or out of a packet?
- Is it mealtime?
- Am I really hungry or just tired or bored?
- Is this extra large pizza with garlic bread worth the weight gain?

Decide what you are going to eat at the start of each day, and you are less likely to submit to the lure of fast foods, to gobble as if your life depended on it or pile your plate till it resembles a small mountain. Not keen on making strategies? How about listening to what your body (really) wants you to eat.

Key Points:

- **Put your cutlery down between mouthfuls**
- **Pay attention to what you are eating**
- **Use a shopping list and stick to it**
- **Cook meals low in added sugar and added fat**
- **Study restaurant menus online before going out**
- **Avoid full board holidays**
- **Plan your daily food intake**

5

THE ART OF INTUITIVE EATING

On a good day you eat three protein rich meals, and reluctantly choose rice rather than pastry. On a bad day you struggle to turn down that second or third slice of chocolate cake and graze all day. You really are trying to eat less and eat better, and even plan ahead to prevent slip ups, but sugary, fatty foods still seems to have the upper hand. So what else can you do to put you, rather than temptation in the driving seat?

Stop bowing down to the food gods, and use your intuition to tune in to what your body actually wants you to eat. It knows when it needs refuelling, if not corrupted by junk foods or influenced by family habits and cultural customs – like leaving your plate clean no matter how much is piled on it, using sweet and fatty foods as a reward, scoffing excessive portions, raiding the fridge at night, eating with the TV on, always having dessert or never refusing seconds.

Spend your day snacking or stuffing yourself to bursting point and you are bound to gain weight. Eat only when you are physically hungry rather than to fill a void and you may find that you have time for all those tasks that you normally put off, like mowing the lawn or knitting a scarf for winter (you wish). Face your emotional pain rather than numbing it with endless trips to the bakery or pub. The pain will still be there in the morning, together with a bigger spare tyre or hangover.

Fixate on food, either by obsessively counting calories or demonising carbohydrate, and you are likely to want to eat more rather than less. Keep it simple: eat three filling meals a day low in added sugar and fat – end of story. Give big name slimming groups a miss. You may make new friends and lose some weight, but they do little to foster the transition to a healthy real food diet because they allow addictive little treats and encourage consumption of commercial diet products.

Purge your kitchen of junk foods; their presence an unhelpful distraction when you are trying to listen to what your body needs. Clear away those biscuits, cakes, savoury snacks, sweets, chocolates and sugary cereals, and make room for basic staples such as tinned tomatoes, dried pulses, dried fruit, pasta, olive oil, wholegrains, herbs and spices. From your fridge chuck the pizzas, ready meals, sausage rolls, puddings, desserts, salad dressing and vegetable oil spread and replace them with meat, fish, eggs, butter, cheese, milk, natural yoghurt, fruit, vegetables, nut butters, nuts, seeds and cooked leftovers.

Defrost the freezer; refilling it with frozen vegetables, potato products, home cooked meals and soups. Okay – you don't really have to chuck stuff; invite your friends over and have a final blow out. Just don't replenish the stocks when they have gone. Your kids will have to get used to it.

Gain confidence in your ability to know what you should

be eating and when to stop. Begin to see food as fuel rather than the answer to all your problems, and before long your favourite snack will cease to taunt you.

Not sure that you want to hear what your body has to say? Treat it like a temple and you may feel less inclined to fill it with junk.

Key Points:

- **Tune into your body**
- **Eat only when physically hungry**
- **Clear your kitchen of processed foods**
- **See food as fuel rather than an answer to all your problems**

6

THE ART OF SELF ESTEEM

Down in the dumps? A chocolate bar, pie or fizzy drink to the rescue, and so begins the slippery slope towards obesity. Instead of using food to cheer yourself up, try finding value in all that life throws at you. It boosts self esteem and makes you less inclined to want to fill your body with mood enhancing foods. Even your dieting hunger pangs can be seen as having an upside – they are an encouraging sign that you are losing weight, so do not rush to stifle them.

Regard your body as a temple and it may prompt you to improve your diet. Yet, what could be more agreeable than a bag of crisps and a cold lager on a hot day? Probably nothing in the short term, however it makes sense to treat your body with the respect it deserves by eating the best food you can afford. Reluctant to give up the foods you love? Full of tasty additives, they make freshly cooked foods seem bland by comparison, but with a little perseverance and the judicious use of a few herbs and spices your taste buds soon adapt.

It's simple: favour real food and eat more protein. Real food is more nutritious than processed and protein is superior to carbohydrates because it is essential for life whereas carbohydrates are not. Protein plays a crucial role in virtually all biological processes and can supply energy if carbohydrates are lacking.

In times past only the king and his nobles ate meat regularly, and the masses had to make do with soup thickened with grains. Protein foods pack such a punch that you only need a little to stay healthy. But upping your intake helps you lose weight and maintain the loss, because they are more filling and harder to assimilate than carbohydrates. Breakfast on a couple of eggs, and include some meat, fish, eggs or cheese at lunch and dinner – no, a pepperoni pizza doesn't count. Some plant foods – Quorn, soya, nuts, seeds and pulses – contain substantial amounts of protein and are a useful replacement for meat.

Vegetables and fruits are carbohydrates, but the amount they contain is small compared to grains because of their high water and fibre content. Rich in vitamins, minerals and super nutrients, they help fight disease and prevent premature ageing. They are an important part of a healthy weight loss diet because vegetables are bulky and fruit helps you wean yourself off refined sugar. Your grandparents knew a thing or two when they served meat with two veg and insisted that an apple a day kept the doctor away. Struggling to eat one vegetable a day and that's tomato ketchup? Let the desire to be slimmer be sufficient incentive to introduce more vegetables to your diet.

Traditionally known as peasant foods, starchy carbohydrates are high in energy and naturally low in fat. They contain varying amounts of protein. Major sources are bread, pasta, potatoes, rice, cereals and pulses. Starchy foods are not strictly necessary, because both protein and fat can be converted into glucose – the body's primary source of fuel, yet they form the basis of diets worldwide because they are plentiful and much cheaper to produce than animal foods. During weight loss, carbohydrates help reduce food cravings.

Refined sugar contains no nutrients other than energy and does not satisfy your appetite like other foods, so use it sparingly and take particular care to avoid drinking copious amounts of liquid sugar in soft drinks and tea and coffee. Before modern times limited amounts of sugar were eaten, obtained from fruits and a little honey.

Natural fat like butter and olive oil contains essential nutrients but only a little is needed for health. Foods like fatty fish, liver, egg yolk and nuts contain more than enough good fats to keep you healthy, so there is no need to add fat or oil to your diet.

Whenever you shop for food or eat out, remind yourself that you are not a dustbin to be filled with rubbish. In time you will grow to appreciate the more complex flavours and firmer consistency of a less processed diet. Respect the beauty of the changing seasons, allowing them to dictate your diet rather than what's on offer at your local supermarket. You know it does not make sense to be eating lettuce in the depths of winter. When it's cold, eat more wholegrains and pulses. Leave salads for warm, summer days.

Don't try to emulate the skinny models you see in fashion magazines. Focusing on unrealistic goals may make you depressed and more likely to reach for the sugar. Take one step at a time and congratulate yourself on your achievements, however small. Practice finding value in all that life throws at you. Soon you start to like yourself more, are motivated to improve your diet, and before long you can do up your buttons without having to breathe in.

Key Points:

- **Find value in adversity**
- **Treat your body like a temple**
- **Protein is king**
- **Only very small amounts of fat are necessary for health**
- **You are not a dustbin to be filled with rubbish**
- **Take one step at a time**

PART TWO

Get Smart

7

FACTS AND FIGURES

Calories

The energy you obtain from your diet is measured in calories. Consume more calories than you need to maintain your weight and the excess is laid down as fat. Create an energy deficit by under eating, and fat is broken down. However calorie counts are no longer considered to be accurate, because they do not take into account the energy required for chewing your meal, moving it through the gut and chemically breaking it down along the way. The most striking inaccuracy is for protein because it is inefficiently metabolised.

The established view is that protein contains 4kcal/g, but it is now thought that the figure for animal protein should be reduced to 2.9kcal/g to allow for the cost of metabolising it. Vegetable protein – soya, other pulses and nuts – is slightly higher in energy. Carbohydrate also contains 4kcal/g, but it is easier to process than protein, making its actual calorie content 3.6kcal/g.

Fat is the most fattening nutrient at 9kcal/g and needs

minimal energy to process it, giving it an amended calorie content of 8.7kcal/g. This makes it three times as fattening as protein and more than twice as fattening as carbohydrates. Although eating lots of fat is the most efficient way to exceed your energy requirements, neither fat nor any other nutrient will make you fat unless you overeat.

The high protein, moderate carbohydrate, low fat diet in Can I Have Chips? is effective because protein is an appetite suppressant and carbohydrates are limited to those that are harder to digest, you therefore take in fewer calories.

Protein

Proteins are made up of amino acids which are needed for cell growth and tissue repair. Depending on which amino acids link together they form enzymes, hormones, muscles, organs and many other tissues in the body. Your body is unable to store excess amino acids for later use and protein must be eaten every day. Gram for gram, protein is the most expensive nutrient.

There are two types of amino acids:

- **Non essential amino acids** which are made by the body
- **Essential amino acids** which cannot be made by the body and must be obtained from food

Animal foods – meat, fish, eggs and dairy products, and certain vegetable foods – soya and Quorn, contain all ten essential amino acids. Other plant foods such as pulses, nuts, seeds and grains, only contain some of them. You can obtain the full complement from a vegetarian diet by eating a variety of plant based foods over the course of a day or two, as different plants lack different amino acids.

It is no coincidence that many ethnic foods combine grains with pulses: Mexican corn and beans, Middle Eastern falafel in pita, Japanese rice and soybeans, Cajun red beans and rice and British baked beans on toast are just a few examples. It is well worth following this tradition. The ideal proportion is approximately two thirds grain to one third pulses. Vegan foods are lower in protein than animal foods, so you need to eat a greater volume of these to obtain the equivalent amount of protein.

Carbohydrate

Need oomph? Grab some carbohydrate; it supplies energy faster than fat. Simple carbohydrates or sugars found in natural foods such as fruit, milk and sweet vegetables do not make you fat as they are diluted by water and often fibre. However the concentrated refined sugars, present in sugary drinks, confectionary, cakes, biscuits and many other processed foods, should be avoided as they lead to energy spikes followed by troughs triggering food cravings.

Complex carbohydrates or starches are found in bread, grains, pulses, potatoes, pasta, bananas and vegetables. They are made up of chains of glucose sugar, but the starchy foods we eat are by no means only energy. They contain varying amounts of protein, fibre, vitamins and minerals and are preferable to simple carbohydrates as a source of fuel.

Want to burn more calories? Eat your starches lightly processed. A muesli bar may contain the same number of calories as a muffin but it is much harder to digest, effectively making it less fattening. See Table 7.1 for foods that are rich in carbohydrate.

Table 7.1
CARBOHYDRATES

Sugars	Starches	Starch/Protein
fruit	vegetables	kidney beans
white sugar	wheat	haricot beans
brown sugar	spelt	chick peas
	rice	black eye peas
glucose fructose	barley	black beans
syrup	oats	butter beans
	corn	split peas
corn syrup	quinoa	lentils
treacle	millet	mung beans
sucrose	potatoes	borlotti beans
malt	yams	white beans
fructose	pasta	soya beans
glucose	bulgur	all other beans
honey	couscous	
golden syrup	bread	
maple syrup	banana	
agave nectar		

Many starchy foods are completely digested but some contain resistant starch, a type of starch that partially resists digestion in the small intestine and becomes available for fermentation by bacteria in the large intestine. Early research indicates that resistant starch can help control weight. It is lower in calories than normal starch – containing around 2.5kcal/g. It suppresses appetite and it increases fat burning by as much as 23% when the intake of resistant starch is only 5.4% of total starch consumed.

Pulses contain the highest percentages of resistant starch, followed by whole, unprocessed grains – particularly barley and corn, firm banana, and cooked and cooled starchy foods such as pasta, rice and potatoes. Baking and deep frying catalyze the formation of resistant starch, making chips and other potato products such as hash browns and croquette potatoes slightly less fattening than their calorie counts suggest. A small daily portion of chips (no more than you can get in a standard mug) as an accompaniment to meat, fish or eggs should not impede weight loss.

Adding more resistant starch does not appear to increase the rate of fat burning or its duration, so a few beans go a long way. Rodents fed resistant starch along with digestible starch maintain smaller fat cells than companions only fed foods high in digestible starch.

Fibre

Studies show that the more fibre you eat the less likely you are to be fat, because foods rich in fibre promote fullness, reduce hunger and are less calorific than low fibre foods.

There are two types of fibre – insoluble and soluble. Insoluble fibre passes through your intestines largely intact, whereas soluble fibre forms a gel when mixed with liquid. Soluble fibre can be broken down in the gut to release energy. This is thought to be around 2kcal/g. See Table 7.2 for foods that are rich in fibre.

Table 7.2
FIBRE RICH FOODS

Soluble Fibre	Insoluble Fibre
oat/oat bran	green beans
dried beans and peas	dark green leafy vegetables
barley	fruit skins
citrus fruit	root vegetable skins
carrots	whole wheat products
flax seed	wheat bran
	corn bran
	seeds & nuts

Many plant based foods rich in fibre also contain resistant starch, a good reason to replace pastries, biscuits and soft drinks with bananas, wholegrains, nuts and seeds.

Fat

All animals and some plants contain fat where it acts as an energy store. Fat is solid at room temperature whereas oil is liquid. There is an inbuilt aversion to overloading on pure fat. When did you last eat a whole pack of butter at one sitting? However, there seems to be no such inner constraints when gobbling fat combined with sugar or flour. This hidden or invisible fat is a major source of fat in the diet.

Our need for fat is extremely low – about one teaspoon a day, which is easily provided by a wholefood diet. Adding extra fat or oil to your meals, or eating food high in added fat is unwise, as fat is three times as fattening as lean protein. In mixed meals, fat is the last nutrient to be used by the body. Alcohol is burnt up first, followed by protein, carbohydrate and fat. It seems that fat is just waiting to get into your fat stores.

Favour small amounts of butter and olive oil, which have been around for centuries, in preference to processed fats and spreads. The effect of long term consumption of these modern fats on health is unknown. These processed fats find their way into convenience foods, takeaways, ready meals, breakfast cereals, cakes, biscuits, confectionary and snacks. All added fats, both natural and processed, increase palatability and make you want to eat more.

There are many natural sources of fat. Cream is made from the butterfat layer skimmed from the top of milk before homogenization. Single cream contains 19g fat per 100ml; double cream contains 48g fat and whipping cream 38g fat. Say no to cream buns, cream cakes and creamy sauces, and resist adding cream to desserts, scones, breakfast cereals, porridge and soups.

Traditional ice cream is made from milk and cream, often combined with fruits or other ingredients and flavours. It provides little nutrition and is high in carbohydrate, mainly sugar and glucose based corn syrup. Artificial flavourings and colourings may be used in addition to, or in replacement of the natural ingredients. Standard ice cream may contain as little as 3g of fat per 100ml but premium ice creams can include as much as 12g. Low fat products are sweeter, to make up for the lack of fat.

Not all ice creams are created equal. The variety you choose has an influence on how much damage it does to your waistline. Eat a large serving of chocolate fudge or cookie dough in a waffle cone, and you may easily consume as many calories as you would on a light lunch. A small scoop of boring vanilla or chocolate, or a fat free sorbet – in a tub of course – is a wiser option. Given that you may be used to eating a much larger amount, you may find this difficult.

The good news is that plain ice cream is less fattening than floury puddings owing to its water content, the bad news is that it's best avoided during weight loss. Stick to fruit and natural yoghurt, you can always suck a frozen banana if the weather is hot.

Think that frozen yoghurt is less fattening than ice cream? It may be low in fat but it is high in sugar, particularly if you succumb to covering it with chocolate sprinkles, mini marshmallows or sugary sauces. Avoid these high sugar (or agave syrup) frozen desserts during weight loss and eat them only occasionally when you reach maintenance.

Food Preparation

In the battle against the bulge, it is not only what you eat that matters. How food is prepared can also make a significant difference.

As a general rule, raw foods are less fattening than cooked foods – 51% percent of raw egg is digested compared to 90% of cooked egg – and wholefoods are less fattening than processed foods. A study in pythons shows that cooking and grinding meat lowers the amount of energy needed to digest a meal by 23%, making a hamburger more fattening than a steak.

Even chewing helps burn (a few) calories, cooked carrots requiring roughly half as many chews as the raw vegetable. So eat your vegetables crispy, your red meat bloody, your starches cold, your food chewy, and give a wide berth to junk foods. With a little stealth and cunning you can eat more of what you like and still lose weight.

Key Points:

- **Food energy is measured in calories**
- **Food contains protein, carbohydrate and fat**
- **Protein is essential for the growth of cells and tissue repair**
- **Carbohydrates and fats are energy rich**
- **Cooking and processing make foods more fattening**

8

WEIGHT LOSS MADE SIMPLE

Live on a regime of fast foods, fatty snacks and soft drinks and you are likely to be carrying excess weight. Studies on populations worldwide confirm this observation. High in added sugar and fat, this pattern of eating is energy rich, very palatable and leads to overconsumption. Want to lose weight long term? Follow a slimming diet that compensates for the natural increase in appetite triggered by dieting.

There is virtually no limit to the amount of fat that you can accumulate. But it is not just fat that causes fat build up – over eat any type of food and you lay down fat. To break it down you must under eat. This is common sense and the scientific evidence is unequivocal. A calorie controlled diet may seem to offer the ideal strategy, but the side effects are hunger, and calorie counting is arduous. A much more effective approach is to manipulate the composition of your diet so that you are not as hungry and you eat less.

Current government nutritional recommendations for a healthy diet are for 15% of your calories to come from protein, 35% from fat and 50% from carbohydrate. But double your protein calories to 30%, reduce your fat intake to 20% and obtain 50% of your calories from carbohydrates that are harder to digest, and you lose weight because you are less hungry. By including carbohydrates in your diet, you avoid a common pitfall of dieting which is a craving for carbohydrate foods.

This method of creating an energy deficit is the basis of the diet in CAN I HAVE CHIPS?. Just eat three protein rich meals a day supplemented with a standard mug (250ml) of cooked starchy food, unlimited vegetables and fresh fruit. It triggers weight loss in all but the smallest builds. Find you are not losing weight? Restrict yourself to half a mug of starchy food. Losing too much? You should be so lucky!

No need to worry that you are eating too much protein. There is no clear evidence that a high protein intake – up to 35% of calories – increases the risk of kidney stones, osteoporosis, cancer or cardiovascular disease, and once you reach phase two (maintenance) you can reduce your intake.

Starchy foods include grains, pasta, pulses and potatoes. They have a reputation for being fattening because they are usually eaten with fat which boosts their energy density. This is the number of calories in a specific amount of food. Low energy density means there are a relatively few calories in a lot of food. High energy density means that there are a lot of calories in a small volume of food. Water and fibre decrease it, whereas fat and sugar increase it. Although nuts are energy dense because they are fatty, they do not seem to prevent weight loss if eaten in moderation as they are high in satisfying protein and their fats are incompletely digested.

Attempt to reduce the volume of food you normally eat and your stomach objects, as the amount of food we like to eat changes little from day to day. But lower the energy density of your meals and you barely notice you are dieting. See Table 8.1 for energy density of carbohydrate based foods.

Table 8.1
ENERGY DENSITY

High	Medium	Low	Very Low
fast foods	bread	grains	green veg
snacks		pulses	fruits
baked goods	breakfast	potatoes	root veg
desserts	cereals	pasta	veg soups
confectionary			
	crispbread		

Key Points:

- **Overeating causes weight gain**
- **Added sugar and added fat lead to overeating**
- **There is no limit to the amount of fat you can accumulate**
- **A high protein, moderate carbohydrate, low fat diet triggers weight loss**
- **High energy density foods are more fattening**
- **Water and fibre decrease energy density**
- **Fat and sugar increase energy density**

9

STARCHES

Starchy carbohydrates found in wholegrains, pulses, pasta and root vegetables, release energy at a steadier pace and keep you feeling fuller longer than easily digested sugary foods. Add some protein, like eggs, cheese, fish, meat or nuts, and you won't feel like snacking between meals. In terms of weight loss not all starchy foods are created equal. The foods you select and the quantities you eat dictate your long term success.

Breakfast Cereals

First thing in the morning after not having eaten for several hours, pick some starchy food to get you going. Listen to your body; eat warm starches like porridge when the weather is cold. In the summer months, breakfast cereals hold more appeal.

Breakfast cereals are made from processed grains. They are usually eaten cold mixed with milk, water or yoghurt. Cereals may be fortified with vitamins. Some are high in fibre but most contain additives and a lot of sugar, particularly those marketed for children. Favour wholegrain cereals with minimal added sugar and no added fat.

Muesli is made from uncooked rolled oats, dried fruit and nuts. It is less easily digested, more filling, and therefore less fattening than processed cereals. Most commercial muesli contains added sugar. Try making your own by mixing muesli base, available from health food stores, with dried fruits, nuts and seeds. Granola is muesli that is toasted with honey and oil to make it crunchy. It is not a slimming breakfast choice as it is high in energy. If you really need to make your oats and muesli taste less like sawdust, simply add some cornflakes or fresh berries.

Porridge is a warm cereal made from rolled oats, ground oatmeal or steel cut oats, and is much more satisfying than muesli and other cold cereals. It is cooked with milk and water in a ratio of one part oats, to two to four parts of liquid. A little salt added towards the end of cooking is often used. Steel cut oats contain the most resistant starch and take longest to cook. Skip the cream and sugar and add some berries instead.

Bread

Traditional bread made from flour and water is the original convenience food; no a croissant does not count as bread. It is easy to scoff large amounts of low fibre white bread, whereas it is much harder to eat fibre rich bread made from coarsely ground grains and seeds. These rough breads contain significant amounts of resistant starch, a type of starch that resists digestion, makes you feel full and boosts your metabolism. Stale bread contains even more. Two medium slices of heavy bread count as one of your three servings of starchy foods a day, so you can have a sandwich for lunch and still lose weight. Help yourself to the world's first fast food, but choose from one of the following types of bread (other than white) to optimize weight loss.

Sourdough

Sourdough bread uses a fermented, batter-like dough starter to make it rise and enhance its flavour. A portion of the sourdough starter is mixed with the bread's ingredients, while the remainder is kept and 'fed' with more flour and water to use in future batches. Sourdough bread is 20% – 30% higher in resistant starch content than bread baked with baker's yeast. Eating sourdough also improves your sugar levels. This is thought to be due to organic acids produced in the bread that delay emptying of the stomach. Most commercial sourdough loaves are made from white flour – a good choice if you can't tolerate a lot of fibre.

Multigrain

Multigrain or seeded bread may contain oats, cracked wheat, buckwheat, barley, millet, rye, sunflower seeds, pumpkin seeds, linseeds or sesame seeds. Raisins and nuts are sometimes added. Most multigrain bread is made with wholemeal flour. Grains and seeds contain significant resistant starch as well as being rich in dietary fibre, protein and essential fatty acids. This makes multigrain bread more wholesome, more satiating and less fattening. Although it does not rise as much, it contains more wheat than the same size loaf of refined bread. You are paying for more grain, more time for production and less air. Wholegrain breads are 50% more filling than white breads.

Pumpernickel

Genuine pumpernickel is a heavy, slightly sweet rye bread traditionally made with coarsely ground rye. It has an exceedingly long baking period. The long slow baking is what gives pumpernickel its dark colour. The bread emerges from the oven deep brown, even black. Like most rye breads, pumpernickel is made with a sourdough starter. Baker's yeast is not useful as a leavening agent for rye bread, as rye does not contain enough gluten. Pumpernickel is about three times as dense as wheat bread. If you like the taste, fulfill your bread ration with pumpernickel. It is almost impossible to overeat.

Stoneground

Until recently all grain was ground between large stones to make flour. Stone grinding ensures that everything in the original grain remains in the finished product. There is no heat buildup, and stoneground flour contains all the naturally occurring vitamins, minerals and micronutrients.

Today most stoneground flour is produced using slow speed steel roller mills which imitate the action of stones. This flour can be listed on the label as stoneground and it is equally nutritious. Stoneground flour contains more resistant starch than normal wholemeal flour. Bread made entirely with 100% stoneground wholegrains will state it on the label. Expect stoneground bread to be heavier, chewier and more expensive. If you don't eat it within a day or two, freeze it until needed.

Wholemeal

Wholemeal flour is produced using modern high speed steel roller mills. Wholemeal bread contains the whole of the product derived from the milling of cleaned wheat, in other words, all the components of the grain – the germ, the bran and the endosperm. It has about 7% fibre, making it less fattening than white bread as it is more filling and less easy to assimilate. Wholemeal flour is finer than stoneground and some of the vitamins are destroyed during the grinding process.

White

White bread is made from flour that contains only the endosperm – the central core of the grain. Grain millers in the nineteenth century discovered that highly refined flour would keep without spoiling for prolonged periods, even before the days of chemical preservatives and refrigeration. Taking the whole grain as 100%, white flour is made by sieving out about 25% of the coarser wheat particles. This includes the germ and the bran. It has about 2% fibre. White bread may contain additives, vitamins and minerals.

Crispbread

Crispbread is a flatbread made from rye flour which is sometimes mixed with other flours. It may contain yeast. Unlike many crackers, traditional crispbread contains no added fat. It contains 50% more resistant starch than ordinary bread owing to the baking process. Varieties include: dark rye crispbread made from wholemeal rye and salt; multigrain rye crispbread topped with a toasted grains, seeds and kernels, and sesame rye crispbread coated with lightly toasted sesame seeds.

Potatoes

Potatoes have a reputation for being fattening. Unfair, as raw potatoes are approximately 75% water and are rated as the most satisfying food per calorie, seven times higher than croissants. Low in energy density, they contain significant amounts of nutrients and have more resistant starch than bread.

Least fattening eaten cold – try serving them with a splash of olive oil, a squeeze of lemon and some spring onion or chives. Roasting and deep frying starchy foods increases their resistant starch and one small daily serving of baked croquette potatoes, hash browns or chips (preferably oven) is unlikely to compromise your weight loss, even though they contain fat.

Look for chips that are simply potatoes and oil, without batter, flour or other additives. Batter coating is designed to add crispness but it adds to the fat and starch content. Chips with additives are tastier, making it harder to limit yourself to just one standard mug. Chunky chips are less fattening than skinny chips because they have less surface area exposed to fat than a thinner chip.

Potato crisps and other savoury snacks contain negligible water making them a high energy density food. Avoid these popular snacks if you hope to lose weight.

Pasta

Like bulgur and couscous, pasta is made from coarsely ground wheat. Less digestible than the finely ground flour used in most bread, eat pasta rather than bread for more effective weight loss. Thick pasta is marginally less fattening than thin pasta. Italy, a nation of pasta lovers, has one of the lowest obesity rates in Europe, but they are more concerned about the quality of the pasta dish than the quantity.

Refrigerating cooked pasta increases its resistant starch content. Pasta is great in summer salads mixed with loads of parsley, olives and chopped tomatoes.

Grains

Grains form the basis of diets worldwide as they are much cheaper to produce than meat. Less digestible and less fattening than flour, grains include wheat, rice, oats, millet, quinoa, barley and corn (maize). A little goes a long way as dry grains absorb water when cooked. Rice is popular because its blandness makes it an ideal accompaniment to foods which have a strong taste. Favour basmati rice, it has the highest level of resistant starch whereas jasmine rice has the lowest. Oats are traditionally eaten as a breakfast food but can also be used in savoury dishes. Easy to cook millet or quinoa add variety to your diet. Include barley in soups, stews or salads. Eat sweetcorn canned or on the cob.

Pulses (beans)

Beans are a good source of energy and they also contain significant amounts of protein, fibre, vitamins and minerals. They possess the highest percentage of protein and resistant starch of any starchy food. Regarded as a food staple, especially in developing countries where they are an important source of protein, they feature prominently on a healthy vegetarian diet.

Whisper the word 'beans' and there may be only one thing that springs to mind and it isn't weight loss. Flatulence is caused by bacteria in the large intestine breaking down food that has not been digested higher up in the intestine. Don't let this minor nuisance get in the way of a slimmer you. Cook beans correctly and it reduces their flatulent effects.

Rich in fibre, beans stabilise blood sugar, even lowering the blood sugar response to food consumed at the next meal. They also contain compounds known as starch blockers which block the action of the enzyme needed to digest starches – good news for dieters. Full of antioxidants, they blunt the inflammatory impact of sugar and refined flour. Not used to beans? Buy a selection of precooked beans and find the ones you prefer. Black beans have the most resistant starch.

Key Points:

- **Starchy carbohydrates keep you feeling fuller longer**
- **Grains, pasta, bread, potatoes and pulses are good sources of starch**
- **Favour low fat, low sugar wholegrain breakfast cereals or porridge**
- **Eat wholegrain breads rather than white**

10

YOUR FIVE A DAY

Not keen on vegetables? Virtually fat free and packed with fibre, they contain plant chemicals that prevent disease. Less fattening eaten raw: peppers, tomatoes, baby corn, mange tout, cucumber, carrots, celery, radishes and fennel are delicious in salads. Eaten before your main course, they reduce your total intake of food at that meal. Salad without dressing is only fit for rabbits, but no need to drown it in oil. In restaurants ask for the dressing on the side and take just a little, or just have vinegar.

During the colder months start your meal with soup – preferably homemade. Vegetable soup, like salad, helps you eat less at mealtimes. A bowl of soup, some sourdough bread and cheese makes a tasty lunch. Virtually any combination of vegetables can be made into a soup by adding them to a base of sweated carrot, celery and onion. Combinations which work well are starchy vegetables, such as parsnips, lentils or potatoes, with one or more watery vegetables such as broccoli, peas, carrot, cauliflower, spinach, mushroom, watercress, pepper, leeks or butternut squash.

Serve at least one vegetable – fresh, frozen or canned –

with your main course, and actually eat them. Steam, sauté in a splash of oil, or bring a little water to the boil and add the vegetables, but don't boil them to death – no need to throw all the nutrients down the plug hole. A scattering of herbs or spices makes tasteless vegetables almost pleasurable. A scraping of butter makes them even nicer. You can even eat them for breakfast. Mushroom and tomato omelette, or cucumber, tomato and pepper sticks with fresh curd cheese, make a change from cornflakes.

Lessen your craving for sugary desserts, puddings and confectionary by eating fresh fruit. Eat the peel where possible as it contains most of the fibre, but make sure you wash it first. Avoid consuming large quantities of sugar rich dried fruit like dates and raisins. A large handful of raisins is equivalent to eating a bunch of fresh grapes in one sitting. Kick your fruit juice habit. You may think it is doing you good, but even unsweetened juices are high in sugar and low in fibre, and liquid sugar does not blunt the appetite. Tomato juice is your best option.

Fruit based desserts have a lower energy density than stodgier puddings, because fruit is fat free and mainly water. Baked apple, stewed cherries with natural yoghurt, fresh figs with cheese, melon and pawpaw, grapes with walnuts, and fruit compote are just some of the many options. Think of fruit as your friend when it comes to achieving a svelte figure and maintaining it. It is as near as you are going to get to the taste of sweetness. Before the introduction of refined sugar, the confectionary of choice for your ancestors was a little honey or a piece of fruit.

Eat the recommended five portions of fruit and vegetables

and you may think that you can reward yourself with a cream cake. It doesn't work quite like that; it is what you don't eat that leads to weight loss.

Key Points:

- **Start your meal with salad (no oil) or vegetable soup**
- **Eat at least one vegetable at lunch and dinner**
- **Eat a piece of fresh fruit for dessert**
- **Limit dried fruit**

11

ME TARZAN

Want to lose that excess fat whilst sparing your precious calorie burning muscle? Eat plenty of protein. At breakfast, replace white toast and jam with eggs on wholegrain toast, or try a ham and potato omelette. Before long you notice that you are no longer ravenous mid morning. Experiment with various protein rich breakfasts until you find the one that keeps you going longest without an attack of the munchies.

At lunch, skip the pasta pot and bag of crisps, and have a cheese, tuna, salmon or turkey sandwich. Vegetarians can combine nuts, seeds or pulses with grains to obtain enough protein. You'll soon wonder what happened to your excess weight.

Meat and Fish

Full of appetite suppressing protein and harder to assimilate than carbohydrate; meat and fish are your allies in the fight against the flab. But eat only protein and you may find yourself low on energy and suffering from constipation, so include some fat free starchy food like rice or potato with your meals. Favour leaner meats such as chicken, turkey, pork, venison and rabbit. Slow cook fattier meats like lamb and duck and discard the fat that is released. Meat is more expensive than starchy foods, so shop around and stock up when the price is low. There is no need to buy the best cuts; cheaper cuts are just as good at filling you up, and so is processed meat.

Fish is an excellent source of protein and is lower in fat than many meats. Haddock, whiting, halibut, plaice and lemon sole, or prawns, scallops and crab; they are all satisfying. No access to fresh or frozen fish? Canned fatty fish such as salmon, tuna, sardines and pilchards is available at most corner shops. Vacuum packed smoked mackerel, salmon and trout is ready to eat. If you can't stand the thought of eating 'real' fish, buy chunky fish fingers or breaded fish fillets that you can cook in the oven.

Milk

Milk is a complex food containing protein, carbohydrate and variable amounts of fat. It is 85% water. Whole milk contains around 3.6g fat per 100ml; semi skimmed milk contains around 1.7g fat, and skimmed is virtually fat free.

Drinking plain milk will not stop you losing weight, but glugging sweetened flavoured milk certainly will. Keep away from those delicious chocolate or strawberry milkshakes and the oversized sweetened offerings topped with cream found at many coffee outlets. These drinks are highly palatable, and whilst you may have difficulty drinking a pint of milk in one sitting – add sugar and cream and down the hatch it goes.

Yoghurt

Made by bacterial fermentation of milk from cows, sheep, goats or buffalo, yoghurt is an excellent replacement for sugary desserts and starchy puddings. But be warned – steer clear of yoghurt products. Most contain thickeners, as well as sugar or artificial sweetener, and flavourings. Even those that purport to contain fruit are high in sugar, as fruit yoghurts are made with jam to extend shelf life. Artificially sweetened yoghurt helps perpetuate your desire for sweetness when you are trying to lose the taste for highly sweetened foods.

Read the label on unsweetened yoghurt and you could be excused for thinking that it contains added sugar. It doesn't, lactose sugar occurs naturally in milk. Like your yoghurt sweet? Buy natural yoghurt and add a teaspoon of jam, honey or maple syrup or better still some berries. The amount of sugar this contributes is negligible compared to that found in a commercial product. You save money and it tastes nicer.

Natural yoghurt is made with whole milk, low fat with semi skimmed, fat free with skimmed, and Greek yoghurt with added cream. Greek yoghurt is rich and creamy, but it still has much less fat than even single cream. So it makes sense to use it as replacement for cream when you reach maintenance; just remember to limit yourself to a pudding spoon or two. If you scoff a whole pot you may as well put a little cream on your dessert.

Cheese

Cheese is the concentrated milk of cows, sheep, goats or

buffalo. It is rich in protein and contains all the essential amino acids. It has a similar amount of protein to meat and fish. It also contains calcium, phosphorous, and vitamins.

Cheese is very nutritious and wonderfully versatile. Where would we be without it? Cheese sandwiches, lasagne, pizza, cheese fondue, cauliflower cheese, cheese salad, cheese and biscuits, cheese sauce, cheeseburgers, cheese and onion crisps, cheese soufflé, cheese and pickle, cheese quiche, the list goes on and on.

But isn't cheese very fattening given that most of its calories come from fat? It depends on how much you eat. It is tasty owing to its high salt content so a little goes a long way. As long as you eat no more than 50g cheese at one sitting it should not impede your weight loss. Your grandparents' generation ate cheese without too much of a problem, but then they did pause for breath between meals and sat down to eat and talked to each other, rather than shovelling in food while watching their favourite soap.

Making cheese sauce? Buy strong cheese rather than mild and you won't need to use so much. Soft cheeses like brie and camembert are creamier than hard cheeses like cheddar, but paradoxically they are lower in fat.

Processed cheese is made from unfermented dairy ingredients and very little real cheese. It contains emulsifiers, salt and food colourings. Many flavours, colours, and textures exist. It is no more fattening than traditional cheese, but the added chemicals make you want to eat more. During weight loss, stick to real cheese, preferably soft cheeses or fresh cheeses. No, you can't have pizza – its energy density is high, it is extremely appetising and a couple of slices are never enough.

Cottage cheese is a low fat, fresh white cheese with a mild flavour. Fromage frais (also known as fromage blanc) is similar to cottage cheese but it is processed until the texture is smooth and free of lumps. Pure fromage frais is virtually fat free, but cream is frequently added to improve the flavour, which increases the fat content. Try fat free fromage frais with berries as a dessert, or add it to savoury dishes.

Ricotta cheese is made from whey, a nutritious liquid that is a byproduct of cheese production. It is creamy white in appearance, slightly sweet in taste and highly perishable. Often used in baking, whole milk ricotta contains 13g fat per 100g. It is a low fat cheese.

Nuts

Technically a large seed, a nut is any large, oily kernel found within a shell that can be eaten. Nuts are highly prized as they are a good vegetarian source of protein and are rich in nutritious oil. They are most healthy in their raw form, because some of the nutrients are lost by heating. Have a delicate stomach? Try soaking nuts in water and little lemon juice for between seven and twenty-four hours before consumption. It improves digestibility.

Nuts include almonds, Brazil nuts, hazelnuts, cashews, macadamia nuts, pecans, pine nuts, pistachio nuts and walnuts. Peanuts are usually regarded as nuts, but technically they are pulses. Although high in fat, studies have found that increased nut consumption does not cause significant weight changes. In fact substituting almonds for carbohydrates in a twenty-four week low calorie diet results in greater weight loss in overweight and obese adults. The reason for this is unclear but could be related to the higher amounts of protein and fibre in nuts, which enhance feelings of fullness and suppress hunger. Or it might be due to increased loss of fat in the faeces due to incomplete mastication.

Nut butters – walnut, cashew, almond and peanut – are delicious spread on sourdough toast. Add nuts to your muesli, porridge and vegetarian dishes. Eat unsalted nuts and you are less likely to eat too many. Crack them yourself and you consume even fewer.

Seeds

Like nuts, seeds are packed with protein but contain more carbohydrate and less fat. Their starches are partially resistant to digestion. Linseeds, pumpkin, sesame and sunflower seeds are a tasty and nutritious addition to breakfast cereals and bread loaves. Try pumpkin seed butter in your sandwiches or on toast.

Tofu

Tofu or bean curd is a vegetarian protein that contains all the essential amino acids. Made by coagulating soy milk and then pressing the resulting curds into soft white blocks, it is low in calories and fat and has very little flavour or smell.

Often marinated in soy sauce, chilli or sesame oil, tofu can be added to savoury or sweet dishes. It can be industrially processed to match the textures and flavours of cheese, eggs, bacon etc.

Quorn

Containing all the essential amino acids, vegetarian Quorn is made from mycoprotein, a member of the fungi (mushroom) family. Cholesterol free and naturally low in fat and calories, it is also high in dietary fibre. Available as ready meals, grills, pieces, sausages, burgers, mince and slices.

Cook Quorn products in your oven, grill, microwave or on the hob, as you would do for meat and poultry. They cook quickly and there is no need to defrost them first.

Pulses

Pulses (beans) are an important part of a vegetarian diet as they contain protein as well as starchy carbohydrate. There are so many varieties of pulse that there is sure to be one that you like, even if it is only the humble baked bean. Canned and cartonned pulses are fat free and ready to eat. Hummus dip made from chick peas is a popular vegetarian standby, but it is high in added fat so favour the low fat versions or make it yourself.

Including some protein at every meal is the key to long term weight loss. Be creative: if you fancy roast chicken for breakfast and beans on toast for dinner, go for it. Your goal is to feel sufficiently full after each meal that you cease to need snacks. See Table 11.1 for protein foods.

Table 11.1
PROTEIN FOODS

Breakfast	Lunch	Dinner
eggs	smoked	steak
sausages	mackerel	pork chop
bacon		fish fillet
kippers	smoked salmon	sea food
	canned tuna	cold cuts
smoked	ham	roast chicken
haddock	omelette	hamburger
	tofu	
cheese	kidney beans	vegetarian
natural yoghurt		sausages
milk	low fat	
baked beans	hummus	Quorn
nuts		

Key Points:

- **Avoid muscle loss when dieting by eating plenty of protein**
- **Animal sources of protein include meat, fish, dairy products and eggs**
- **Vegetable sources of protein include nuts, seeds, pulses, tofu and Quorn**

12

LIQUID REFRESHMENTS

Energy drinks, flavoured lattes, fruit juice or bog standard fizzy cola; drink these regularly and don't expect to lose weight. Believe their wonderful marketing claims and you might be persuaded to include them into your daily diet. Treat liquid calories as a waste of space; down the hatch in a flash you barely notice what is passing your lips.

Soft Drinks

There is a close parallel between the dramatic increase in the consumption of sugar sweetened drinks in the last thirty years and the obesity epidemic in the United States, which is now spreading elsewhere. Several large studies have demonstrated the connection. Eat sugar in solid form as jelly beans and you are likely to reduce food intake later, but drink sugary sodas and they won't spoil your appetite. Given that you may be drinking several daily, now is the time to stop the pop.

But what about pure fruit juice, surely that must be okay? Sorry, but no. Although it is a natural fruit product, fruit juice contains almost as much sugar as fizzy drinks. No one is denying you fresh fruit but eat it whole, preferably including the skin if it is edible. It is harder to eat a fresh apple replete with fibre than downing a large juice which may contain several fruits. It is not all doom and gloom though; drink tomato or carrot juice or try sparkling water flavoured with a squeeze of fresh lemon or lime. Just don't add sugar.

Energy Drinks

Energy drinks claim to promote weight loss and improve stamina, athletic performance and concentration. The common ingredient in most energy drinks is the stimulant caffeine – about three times the amount as cola. Although in the short term caffeine has a beneficial effect on energy metabolism, in the long term its effect on energy balance and body weight are unclear.

The stimulating effect of energy drinks is not only derived from caffeine, but also from a variety of other stimulants such as ginseng, taurine, guarana and B complex vitamins. Many brands offer artificially sweetened 'diet' versions. Non diet versions of energy drinks contain between six and twelve teaspoons of sugar per can. The high sugar content makes them not only ineffective in promoting weight loss but also a cause of weight gain.

Tea and Coffee

Weaning yourself off sugary tea and coffee is an important first step towards weight loss. But what if your favourite drink is white chocolate or peppermint mocha topped with whipped cream and chocolate curls? These liquid desserts are not compatible with dieting owing to the large amount of sugar and fat they contain. You would be better off having a solid dessert, as it is more likely to blunt your appetite.

Diet Drinks

Imbibing diet drinks rather than regular sugared varieties might seem to be a sensible idea, but is it really? Although some human studies suggest that sugar substitutes help with short term weight loss, an equal number suggest they don't. They are at least 200 times as sweet as sugar, and that is a potent stimulus for a sweet tooth. If artificial sweeteners increase your cravings for sweet food, they become counterproductive. The calories they take out of your diet are apt to sneak back in later when you want a larger or sweeter dessert to feel satisfied.

See Table 12.1 for drinks you are allowed and those that are best avoided.

Table 12.1
DRINKS

Permitted	Not Permitted
water	sweetened coffee
coffee	coffee with cream
tea	sweetened tea
milk	energy drinks
herb tea	fizzy drinks
fruit tea	soft drinks
sparkling water	fruit juice
soda water	fruit drinks
vegetable juice	diet drinks
tomato juice	milk shakes
carrot juice	

Key Points:

- **Sugar sweetened drink consumption is linked to obesity**
- **Liquid sugar doesn't spoil your appetite**
- **Energy drinks rich in sugar promote weight gain**
- **Diet drinks are a stimulus for a sweet tooth**

13

ALCOHOL
THE FOURTH MACRONUTRIENT

Desperate to lose that beer belly or lardy arse but not planning to give up your lads' night out, girls' night in, or solitary nightcap? Well you've got to relax somehow, and it is legal. Surely there is a way you can carry on your drinking habit and still lose weight. The French manage to stay relatively slim whilst drinking copious amounts of wine, so it must be possible.

Often called the fourth macronutrient, alcohol is a significant energy source containing 7kcal/g and no other nutrients. Alcohol is the priority fuel for your body. Drink alcohol while you eat, and it increases the likelihood of your food ending up as fat. On the plus side, the cost of metabolising it is high – at 20% to 30%.

Ferment fruits, cereals and even some vegetables and leaves and you end up with alcohol – and no, it doesn't count as one of your five a day. During fermentation, yeast eats up the carbohydrates. Whatever sugar is left contributes to the carbohydrate in the beverage. Dry wine has little residual sugar, whereas sweet wine and beer has more. Some liqueurs such as Amaretto or Crème de Menthe have sugar added.

Non distilled beverages – wine, beer and cider – are less potent than distilled drinks – aperitifs, whiskies, liqueurs, rum and vodka. However, when it comes to your waistline, your choice of drink is less important than the quantity you imbibe.

Not only is alcohol calorific – particularly sweetened drinks – but it also inhibits fat breakdown and induces fat storage. Drink moderately – up to two glasses of wine a day – and studies show you compensate by eating less and don't gain weight. Drink heavily, however, and you end up eating more because it loosens inhibitions. What may be hard to resist when sober may be nigh on impossible when drunk. Regular drinking sessions, bar snacks and the statutory after pub curry can scupper your chances of weight loss. But gradually reduce your pub visits, avoid the worst of the late night takeaways, and you are in with a chance of success despite your alcohol habit.

Take extra care if you like a mixer with your alcohol. Be it cola, tonic, orange juice, lemonade or cordial, they are little more than sugar. As an alternative, try soda water, sparkling water or a squeeze of fresh lemon. Some alcoholic drinks known as alcopops are already mixed. Their sugar content makes them highly palatable making you less conscious of how much you are drinking.

Bar Snacks

Have a drink, and a nibble is never far behind. Cunningly most bar snacks are salty, making you thirsty as well as fat. If you want a snack, munch some peanuts. They may be high in fat but they contain as much protein as meat. Or eat olives – nutritious and harder to overeat.

Post Pub Meals

Going out drinking? Have a meal first. You drink less and may not be as keen on a midnight feast. Too drunk to care what you consume as you wind your way home? Try planning your post pub meal while sober. Say no to anything swimming in grease – yes it's the nation's favourite dish, chicken tikka masala. Go for the mixed grill instead. At your local chippie, order a portion of fish or meat with a small serving of chips.

Kebab houses are probably your best bet. That's a kebab made from real pieces of meat in pita bread with salad and no oil, not the infamous doner consisting of unidentified bits of meat reheated numerous times so that it becomes a public health hazard. If a hangover doesn't floor you the next day, your doner probably will. See Table 13.1 for drinking guidelines.

Table 13.1
DRINKING GUIDELINES

Permitted	Not Permitted
moderate drinking	binge drinking
wine/beer/cider/spirits	alcopops
peanuts/olives	sweetened mixer drinks
pre pub eating	savoury snacks
	post pub takeaways

Key Points:

- Alcohol is a significant energy source
- Alcohol inhibits fat breakdown and increases fat storage
- Mixer drinks contain added sugar
- Eat a meal before going drinking
- Choose peanuts or olives as bar snacks

PART THREE

Get Real

14

THE DIET

Not sure that you need to lose weight? After all, most of your friends have muffin tops or beer bellies. Try weighing yourself, or better still work out your body mass index. A mass of twenty-five to thirty says you are overweight and above thirty obese. Need convincing? Find a full length mirror and take a good look at yourself naked; the answer should be apparent.

Fast foods, soft drinks and snacks; if this is all you consume it is not surprising that you are carrying excess pounds. Want to be slimmer? Switch to a more wholesome diet and eat less. Slimming groups are popular because they provide companionship and support, but they do little to address the root cause of your predicament – an addiction to sugary, fatty food. This explains why their long term success rates are abysmal. Yes, they keep quiet about these statistics on their marketing material.

Follow a low fat diet – a popular strategy – and you are sure to lose weight because fat is rich in energy, but you are unlikely to find a long term solution to your weight problems. Food is less appetising, cooking is a chore, fat is replaced with sugars and refined starches, and before long you are stuffing yourself with all your old standbys. A more sustainable approach is to stop eating energy dense sugary and fatty foods, replacing them with proteins and harder to digest carbohydrates that suppress the appetite and reduce food cravings.

Buying real food need not break the bank. More expensive than processed, but you save serious dosh by cutting out snacks. No need to splash out on the most costly foods either. Your grandparents' generation managed to survive, and actually thrived without avocado pears, mangoes, designer cheeses, mangetout peas and the best cuts of meat, yet they remained slim, at least until well past middle age when metabolism naturally slows and activity levels decline. They ate eggs, cheese, corned beef, sausages, ham, liver, kidneys, vegetables, cereals, bread, potatoes, apples, pears, canned fruit, custard, dry biscuits, jelly and puddings. Wine drinking at home was rare and an expensive treat. Snacking was seen as ruining your appetite. If they did snack it was on an apple, a slice of bread and butter, a glass of milk, or a cup of tea with a plain biscuit.

Embark on a regime of three meals a day of real food containing plenty of protein, cut out snacks and sugary drinks, and expect to see quick weight loss which tapers off as you approach a healthy weight. If you have post menopausal weight gain caused by hormonal changes, you may find that you need to restrict yourself to half a mug of starch per meal and up your protein intake before you start losing weight. Slimming down too fast – eat more, but don't be tempted to supplement your daily regime with added sugar or fat.

How rapidly you lose weight depends on your starting

weight. The heavier you are, the easier it is, as the disparity between what you currently eat and what is permitted on the diet is greater. Anticipate dropping about five pounds in the first week, tapering off in subsequent weeks. Make your goal realistic and expect blips, usually caused by nibbling surreptitious snacks and drinking one too many glasses of wine.

Reached your goal or run out of steam? Proceed to maintenance. Maintain your lower weight for at least twelve weeks, before returning to another bout of weight loss if needed. Be warned, rush into the diet without taking on board the mental changes described at the beginning of the book and don't be surprised that you find it too challenging. But eat less, eat better, adopt some cunning weight loss strategies, eat intuitively, and develop your self esteem, and there is little to hold you back from the body you desire.

PROHIBITED FOODS

Prohibited foods are those that contain significant amounts of added sugar, added fat or both, ruling out sugar sweetened drinks and most processed foods. These palatable foods encourage overeating, and weight gain is the result. During phase one – weight loss – the fewer of these you eat the quicker you lose weight. Remember that it is eating and drinking too much that makes you fat, not any specific food.

Added Sugars

Table sugar or sucrose is the most common added sugar in our diet, but there are many other sugars – their names often ending with 'ose' that are used to sweeten food and drink. Even savoury processed foods usually contain added sugar, and it is hard to avoid completely unless you cook food from scratch.

The first item mentioned on an ingredient list is the most abundant, so manufacturers sometimes divide added sugar into multiple aliases in order to make a product appear less sweet than it actually is. See Table 14.1 for a list of common sugars.

Table 14.1
SUGARS

sucrose
glucose
maltose
honey
treacle
maple syrup
malt
molasses
golden syrup
corn syrup
agave nectar
fructose
glucose fructose syrup

Added Fats

Fat makes food taste better but it is high in energy. Avoid junk foods which are high in fat and restrict yourself to small portions of real foods containing added fat such as chips or roast potatoes. Learn to prepare your meals with minimal added fat. There is plenty of fat in foods such as meat, cheese, eggs, fatty fish, nuts and seeds so there is no possibility of becoming deficient. See Table 14.2 for a list of fats.

Table 14.2 **FATS**
butter
cream
lard
margarine
oil
vegetable oil spreads
salad dressing

Carb/Fat Combos

Chew a lump of fat and you are unlikely to want seconds. Yet mix it with flour or sugar and it becomes irresistible. Give these sweet or savoury carb/fat combos a miss; just one bite leads to another and then another. See Table 14.3 for carb/fat combos.

Table 14.3
CARB/FAT COMBOS

Sweet	Savoury
pastries	Cornish pasties
croissants	samosas
cupcakes	spring rolls
muffins	sausage rolls
biscuits	pies
cakes	garlic bread
doughnuts	crackers
mousse	savoury snacks
puddings	cheese straws
desserts	buttered popcorn
ice cream	
toffee	
chocolate bars	
toffee popcorn	

PERMITTED FOODS

Permitted foods are those that are natural or only minimally processed. They help you lose weight because they are filling and are low in added sugar and fat. They may contain natural sugar and fat, but the quantities are small compared to the amounts found in processed foods. In communities where only real foods are eaten, obesity is rare.

During weight loss, most processed foods found at your local supermarket must be off limits, but there is no need to panic. Look carefully and you will notice real food – meat and fish (fresh, frozen, canned, smoked or cured), wholegrains, pulses, halfway decent bread, dairy products, and fruits and vegetables. See Table 14.4 for permitted foods.

Table 14.4
PERMITTED FOODS

Protein	Starchy Carbohydrates
meat	heavy bread
fish	pulses (beans)
eggs	banana
cheese	potato
milk	sweet potato
yoghurt	yam
nuts (excluding chestnut)	plantain
peanut butter	rice
almond butter	oats
cashew butter	whole wheat
walnut butter	pasta
pumpkin seed butter	couscous
soya products	bulgur wheat
Quorn products	millet
pulses (beans)*	quinoa
	spelt
	barley
	corn (maize)
	muesli
	low sugar breakfast cereals
*pulses contain protein	porridge
and starch	chestnut

Table 14.4
PERMITTED FOODS

Fruits	Vegetables
pear	cabbage
plum	kale
apple	carrot
orange	beetroot
lemon	peas
grapefruit	leek
grapes	turnip
cherry	onion
mango	parsnip
melon	garlic
berries	swede
kiwi fruit	broccoli
peach	mushrooms
nectarine	celery
apricot	green beans
pineapple	mange tout
guava	broad beans
fig	cauliflower
coconut	squash
	bell pepper
	artichoke
	lettuce
	avocado
	tomato

Getting Started

Throw yourself headlong into any new diet and you risk reversing out just as rapidly. Find eating real food an alien concept? Take it slowly and save yourself some serious discombobulation. Sugar in tea and coffee is a waste of space. Go cold turkey or cut down one teaspoon at a time over the course of a week or two. Within days sweetened hot drinks will taste too sweet. If you must have something sugary from time to time, make it something solid that takes longer to eat.

Next give up soft drinks. Sugar sweetened drink consumption is strongly associated with obesity. Think fruit juice is better for you as it contains vitamins? A glass of juice contains about the same amount of sugar as a fizzy drink. Diet drinks are not the solution. They may contain zero calories but their sweet taste does not help you lose the taste for sugar. Drink water instead.

Having difficulty getting through your day without a snack? Sweet or savoury, expensive or cheap, snack on foods containing added sugar and fat and you are soon hungry again. Eat three filling meals a day of real food and it won't be hunger that drives you to eat between meals. If you really can't wait until your next meal; have an orange or apple, or a few nuts and seeds until you acquire the habit of not eating between meals. A small square of 70% or 85% plain dark chocolate after lunch and dinner helps satisfy a sweet tooth, as long as you have the willpower to stop after a small piece. No, you can't have a mini Mars bar – too sweet and too moreish.

Given up snacks? Now ditch the cotton wool – I mean

mass produced bread, particularly white. Denser loaves are filling, and eating less is what you are aiming for. Heavy bread is more difficult to digest – in one end and out the other. Look out for wholegrain or seeded, stoneground, sourdough or pumpernickel. Discover a good loaf? Stick some in the freezer.

Practise applying heat to raw food, otherwise known as cooking. Those wonderful labour saving ready meals and takeaways are tempting when you have a family to feed or are in a rush, but most are incompatible with weight loss. Low fat 'diet' meals are not the solution as sugars and starches replace fats, one meal is never enough to fill you up, and eating more than one defeats the purpose of dieting.

Replace readymade desserts with fruit and natural yoghurt, less fattening and more refreshing. Reluctant to give up your social life as you know it, but are up for cutting down on alcohol consumption? Try spending fewer nights out boozing. This strategy is more successful than drinking mineral water at the pub, listening to your mates poking fun at you whilst downing pint after pint.

Fed up of rehearsing and ready to take the plunge? Start with day one and the rest will follow seamlessly. Before long you begin to wonder what took you so long. Expect your progress to be without blips and you are likely to give up and go back to your old eating habits. But treat each day as a fresh start and success is yours for the taking.

Key Points:

- **Eat three protein rich meals a day**

- Limit added sugar and added fat
- Give up sugary drinks
- No snacking between meals
- Cut back on alcohol

15

FINDING YOUR FATNESS TYPE

Acknowledge that you are overweight, and you are half way to achieving the body you desire. Understand why you overeat and you increase your chances of success.

Work out your fatness type before embarking on phase one – weight loss. Then when tempted by that cold pint of beer or warm chocolate brownie mutter the affirmation that suits you best.

Sleeping Beauty Type

You rarely think about your size. You are unlikely to diet unless your partner forces you to look at yourself in a full length mirror. Blissful ignorance is your motto.

- *I choose to wake up and deal with my excess weight*

Routine Type

You know what foods you like and you like what you know. You don't intend to change your habits of a lifetime even if it means staying fat. You hate having your routine upset.

- *I choose to welcome new eating habits*

Greedy Type

Scoffing is your middle name. You polish off a 100g bar of chocolate in one sitting, or drink seven pints of lager at the pub. Doing without is not your style.

- *I choose to behave like a human being rather than a pig*

Ostrich Type

You inhale your food, wipe your plate clean, load your shopping basket with crisps and desserts, snack all day and raid the fridge at night. Although everyone else can see why you are fat, you can't. What you don't see can't harm you, can it?

- *I choose to see my fattening eating habits*

Hard of Hearing Type

You have no idea what to eat or how much. If it's there you eat it.

- *I choose to hear what my body wants me to eat and when it tells me to stop*

Dustbin Type

You are out of your comfort zone. You eat fatty snacks to quell the unease. You feel bad so you prefer rubbish.

- *I am special and deserve the best*

16

PHASE ONE

Forearmed with knowledge of the enemy, you are ready to embark on phase one. It is protein rich, low in added sugar and fat, and designed to trigger quick weight loss. It is simple to follow and it works. You are no longer destined to spend every waking minute obsessing about food. Look on the bright side, starchy carbohydrates and fruits are permitted, you are even encouraged to include them, as they help to offset the increase in hunger and food cravings induced by dieting. It may be monotonous but it is not harsh.

UNDERSTANDING THE PLAN

You don't need commercial diet products, you don't need to count calories, you don't need a degree in nutrition. You do need to adopt new eating habits, you do need to build up your self esteem, you do need to know which foods make you fat.

Base your meals on a normal serving of protein and one standard mug (250ml) of cooked starchy food. Vegetables and whole fresh fruit (excluding bananas) eaten at mealtimes are unlimited.

Don't know what a normal serving of protein looks like? It is a typical restaurant portion: a chicken breast but not a whole chicken, a few slices of roast lamb but not the whole leg, a handful of nuts but not a whole pack, a medium steak, an egg or two, a 50g piece of cheese or half a pint of milk.

One standard mug of cooked starchy food is equivalent to 50g of uncooked grain, 65g dried pasta, one banana, four crispbread or two medium slices of bread. Aim to feel satisfied after a meal, not stuffed. Find these quantities too much? Eat less as long as you are not tempted to snack between meals. Still hungry – eat more protein and vegetables.

Phase one is nutritionally complete, but no diet is sustainable for long without the inclusion of some flour, added sugar and added fat. Are chips your weakness? A little of what you fancy does you good if it helps you stick to the diet. Chips fill you up and are less fattening than pastry or biscuits because they contain water. Don't like chips? Treat yourself to one square of plain dark chocolate (70% or 85%) after lunch and dinner. You may also drink one alcoholic drink a day. Find it hard limiting yourself to one? Then it is better to abstain completely until you have reached your goal weight. See Table 16.1 for daily permitted extras.

Table 16.1
DAILY PERMITTED EXTRAS

3 tsp flour
3 tsp sugar, honey, maple syrup or jam
4 level tsp butter, oil or mayonnaise
Either one small serving chips, roast potatoes or hash browns **or** two squares plain dark chocolate
125ml glass wine or ½ pint beer

DO

- Eat three meals a day
- Eat a normal serving of protein at every meal
- Eat one standard mug (250ml) of cooked starchy food or equivalent at every meal
- Eat vegetables and fruit

DON'T

- Exceed amounts of daily permitted extras
- Eat fast foods
- Eat junk foods
- Skip meals
- Drink fruit juice or sugary drinks
- Eat between meals
- Eat during the night
- Drink more than one alcoholic drink a day

BREAKFAST

1 normal serving protein + 1 standard mug cooked starchy food + fruit/vegetables

Start your day with a filling breakfast containing protein and carbohydrate. Missing breakfast increases the production of appetite stimulating hormones which lead to daytime overeating. A banana, a few nuts and an apple, or a slice of cheese or meat with heavy bread and an orange, are the quickest breakfasts on the planet, so there is no excuse. Chocolate biscuits or crisps washed down by cola do not count as breakfast.

Create your own breakfast (Table 16.2) by picking a protein food and a starchy food. Pulses contain both protein and starch. Add some fruit or vegetables if you wish. Alternatively, try one of the phase one suggested breakfasts (Table 16.3). After breakfast don't eat until lunchtime.

Table 16.2
CREATE YOUR OWN BREAKFAST

Pick a protein food	Pick a starchy food	Pick fruit/vegetables
boiled eggs	porridge	any (except banana or potato)
fried eggs	noodles	
scrambled eggs	chips	
omelette	1 banana	
kippers	2 hash browns	
ham	baked beans	
bacon		
2 sausages	medium baked potato	
tofu		
baked beans		
nut/seed butter	2 medium slices bread★	
natural yoghurt		
milk		
cheese (50g)	unsweetened muesli	
nuts/seeds (small handful)	low fat, low sugar breakfast cereal	

★ sourdough, stoneground, pumpernickel or wholegrain/seeded

Drinks – unsweetened tea, coffee, herb or fruit tea, milk or water

Table 16.3 PHASE ONE SUGGESTED BREAKFASTS	
Monday	muesli with natural yoghurt, fresh fruit or egg, bacon, mushrooms, tomato and 2 hash browns
Tuesday	miso soup with noodles, spring onion and shredded chicken or porridge with pumpkin/sunflower seeds, raspberries
Wednesday	toast with nut/seed butter, 2 prunes or dried figs or pumpernickel bread with ham and mustard, cherries
Thursday	baked beans on toast, blueberries or cornflakes, 10 hazelnuts, raisins and milk
Friday	medium baked potato, 50g grated cheese, apple or 2 fried eggs and chips, satsuma

Saturday	kippers, tomato and sourdough bread or 30g cheese, grapes, banana and 6 brazil nuts
Sunday	low sugar/fat cereal, flaked almonds, strawberries and milk or scrambled eggs, mushrooms and wholegrain toast

Drinks – unsweetened tea, coffee, herb or fruit tea, milk or water

LUNCH

1 normal serving protein + 1 standard mug cooked starchy food + fruit/vegetables

Create your own lunch (Table 16.4), pick one of the phase one suggested lunches (Table 16.5) or have a sandwich. Pulses (beans) contain both protein and starch. Do not exceed permitted daily amounts of flour, fat and sugar. After lunch, don't eat until dinner.

Table 16.4
CREATE YOUR OWN LUNCH

Pick a protein food	**Pick a starchy food**	**Pick fruit/vegetables**
cold meats	pasta	any (except
roast chicken	chips	banana or
kebab	grains	potato)
fish fingers	potatoes	
breaded fish	pulses (beans)	
canned tuna	sweetcorn	
seafood	banana	
smoked salmon	2 slices bread★	
canned salmon		
Quorn	4 slices	
tofu	wholegrain	
cheese (50g)	crispbread	
nuts (small handful)		
pulses (beans)		

★ sourdough, stoneground, pumpernickel or wholegrain/ seeded

Drinks – unsweetened tea, coffee, herb or fruit tea, or water

Table 16.5 PHASE ONE SUGGESTED LUNCHES	
Monday	salmon/tuna, spring onion, cucumber and new potatoes
Tuesday	medium baked sweet potato, 50g grated cheese and mixed salad (no oil)
Wednesday	prawn salad, 30g cheese and crispbread
Thursday	baked chunky fish fingers or breaded fish fillet, green beans and carrots
Friday	basmati rice, crushed hazelnuts and peas
Saturday	ham, chips and salad (no oil)
Sunday	roast chicken, millet and vegetables

Drinks – unsweetened tea, coffee, herb or fruit tea, or water
Dessert – diced fruit with 2 pudding spoons natural yoghurt

Sandwiches

Where would we be without our favourite lunchtime sandwich? Possibly a lot thinner. High in added fat, surely sandwich eating is hard to reconcile with weight loss? But all is not lost. You can still tuck into a shop bought sandwich and shed the pounds as long as you pick the best available bread, a protein rich filling, and only eat one round. Look for sandwiches with less than 10g fat per pack, and avoid the crisps and soft drink that often accompany them.

Having a freshly prepared sandwich? Make it yourself, or order a granary or wholemeal bread sandwich with a scraping of mayo or butter. Round off your sandwich meal with an apple and it should keep you going till dinner.

DINNER

Starter (optional) + main course + fruit

Create your own dinner by selecting a starter, followed by a main course (Table 16.6), or try one of the phase one suggested dinners (Table 16.7). No snacking after dinner.

Starters

mixed salad
vegetable soup (no cream)
avocado and tomato salad (no oil)
smoked salmon
asparagus spears
half grapefruit (no sugar)

Table 16.6
PHASE ONE MAIN COURSES

Pick a protein food	Pick a starchy food	Pick vegetables
roast chicken	mashed potato	any (except potato)
roast pork	chips	
lamb kebab	roast potato	
prawns	roast parsnip	
scallops	millet	
steak	quinoa	
turkey strips	basmati rice	
3 sausages	couscous	
tofu	pulses	
Quorn	pasta	
nuts	yam	
pulses (beans)	2 slices bread★	
baked fish		
cheese (50g)		

★ sourdough, stoneground, pumpernickel or wholegrain/seeded

Drinks – unsweetened tea, coffee, herb or fruit tea, water, one small glass wine or half pint beer
Dessert – fruit

Table 16.7 PHASE ONE SUGGESTED DINNERS	
Monday	lentil dal, basmati rice and vegetables
Tuesday	braised beef, carrots, shredded cabbage and pasta
Wednesday	onion and potato omelette, and sweetcorn
Thursday	sausage, egg, chips, lettuce (no oil) and tomato
Friday	grilled fish fillet, mashed potato and leeks
Saturday	tofu, quinoa, peppers, onions and tomatoes
Sunday	homemade Brussel sprouts and chestnut soup and bread

Drinks – unsweetened tea, coffee, fruit or herb tea, water, one small glass wine or half pint beer

Dessert – fruit

Dining Out

It is much easier to lose weight if you cook your meals from scratch, but just possible when you eat out, as long as you can visualise how much starchy food you can squash into a standard mug and have the willpower to order the lower fat options – there must be some! Find the portions too big? If you haven't managed to compensate by eating less at lunchtime, skip the starter or share a main course.

Limit eating out to once a week during phase one, as your resolve is bound to falter when you see your companions scoffing soft white bread, creamy sauces and yummy desserts. Wherever you decide to dine, vary your carbohydrates. Choose bread or cereal for breakfast and potatoes for lunch, favour pulses or pasta at dinner and don't forget to eat your vegetables.

Condiments, Herbs and Spices

Fast foods are appealing partly because they are tasty. Pep up your homemade meals with condiments, herbs and spices (Table 16.8) to help you make the transition to healthier fare. Some condiments are high in sugar and must be counted as part of your permitted daily sugar rations. Avoid fat laden cooking sauces – a small amount is never enough.

Table 16.8
CONDIMENTS, HERBS AND SPICES

Condiments	Herbs	Spices
vinegar	thyme	salt
soy sauce	oregano	pepper
teriyaki sauce	marjoram	cumin
tomato sauce	parsley	chilli
relish	coriander	turmeric
mustard	basil	cinnamon
chilli sauce	dill	vanilla
black bean	rosemary	cloves
mango chutney	sage	nutmeg
cranberry sauce	mint	mace
Worcester sauce	chives	five spice
brown sauce	bay	curry
pesto		paprika
		garlic
		ginger
		star anise

Damage Limitation

Phase one is a doddle – or is it? Your train home is delayed; you buy a bag of sweets from a vending machine. Slumped in front of the TV after your wholesome evening meal, a stray walnut whip slips into your mouth. At the local with your pals, there's no way you are drinking mineral water or saying no to a late night curry.

Given in to temptation? Make amends later. Your lapse is at breakfast, you have the rest of the day to be abstemious. But slip up in the evening when social activity is at its peak and you must compensate the following day.

Guzzled like a pig today? Nibble like a rabbit tomorrow on carrots and lettuce, or take some prunes and hope they do the trick. Don't beat yourself up about your occasional lapses. Life's too short to deny yourself all earthly pleasures. After all you didn't train to be a monk (or nun).

17

PHASE TWO

You reach your goal or shed some poundage and breathe a sigh of relief. Hooray, back to eating normally. Not so fast – don't expect to eat 'like you used to'. The new slimmer you doesn't need as much food as the heavier version. Want to stay slim? Simple – follow the weight maintenance plan for at least six months. It takes this long for ghrelin, the appetite stimulating hormone that is triggered by weight loss, to return to normal. This is why rigid, faddy diets that you can't stick to result in rebound weight gain, plus a bit more for luck.

Phase two – weight maintenance, is not as strict as phase one – weight loss. It is a question of degree, but continue to do your best to avoid food and drink containing added sugar or added fat. This does not mean you can't eat any sugar or fat. As long as they are an integral part of real food and you don't eat huge portions, you can include them in your diet. Natural sugars are present in fruit, and natural fat is found in meat, fish, dairy, nuts and seeds.

Phase two is about learning to make good food choices in your daily life. Home cooked meals, restaurant meals or convenience foods; take your pick. It is what they don't contain that matters. You no longer need to eat as much protein, now that you are not actively trying to lose weight, but resist the temptation to cut back on vegetables, they help fill you up. Step on the scales regularly, their instant feedback is a potent reminder to stay on the straight and narrow.

Maintaining your lower weight in a world where eating fast foods is the norm, is not about following a strict set of rules. It is a complex dance where good days mingle with bad, and a fundamentalist approach can only lead to failure. It is so challenging that over 95% of dieters are unable to achieve it. But carry on eating real foods and avoiding processed foods, and an end to yo-yo dieting is in sight.

Staying slim is a veritable minefield as there is a mismatch between ever growing portion sizes and your need for sustenance. Consume a takeaway or even a restaurant meal that provides you with enough fuel for two meals, and it is one step forward and two steps back. You are designed to eat three times a day and not require food at night.

What you eat at mealtimes is only the tip of the iceberg. Does it matter if your evening meal is baked potato and grated cheese; chicken, rice and peas, or beans on toast eaten in moderation? Not in the grand scheme of your weight it doesn't. They all contain protein and are low in added sugar and added fat. It is what you eat and drink between meals that make the difference between staying the same weight and seeing it creep up again.

Begin to trust in your ability to know when you have eaten enough for one day. You cannot go back to your old way of eating; that is if your desire to stay trim is greater than the urge to stuff yourself with sugary treats.

Rediscover your social life and stop being a 'party pooper'. Give up your favourite foods for a while, fair enough, but a lifetime without those buttery croissants, tasty sausage rolls, stress busting chocolate or flavoursome crisps is never going to happen. It's not in your nature to forgo life's little pleasures. Try eating your favourite snack occasionally rather than every day, or just have a nibble, and you shouldn't have too much of a problem keeping your weight stable.

Practise eating out without throwing caution to the wind. Experiment with new foods – it increases your chance of long term success. If you've never eaten natural yoghurt, pulses or fatty fish, now is the time to start.

Welcome to the real world where fast foods lurk at every corner. Deal with it; it is not going to change any time soon. Include some readymade foods if it makes your life easier – the difficulty is finding ones that are not loaded with added sugar and added fat. Enjoy small servings of less fattening homemade desserts (see chapter 22) and feel free to drink in moderation.

Choosing ready meals or precooked dishes that do not expand your waistline is a minefield for the uninitiated. If you can't work out what is in your ready meal, don't eat it. Seek out meals rich in protein. This is difficult because animal protein is expensive. What they lack in protein they gain in cheap flour and fat. Shop bought or restaurant made desserts and puddings are by their very nature highly calorific. The fewer of these you eat the better.

Cook battered or breaded foods like fish fingers or fish fillets in the oven without oil, rather than frying them which increases the fat content. If the pack says it serves two people, you can't scoff it all yourself without expecting to put on weight. Starchy foods eaten at every meal help you avoid between meal munchies. Choose from potatoes, grains, pasta or pulses, or a mixture of these. At dinnertime, have soup or salad to start, a main course and a small portion of homemade dessert (see Chapter 22).

DO

- Try new foods
- Include convenience foods
- Limit added sugar and added fat
- Eat three meals a day
- Eat some protein at every meal
- Eat vegetables
- Eat fruit

DON'T

- Drink fruit juice, soft drinks or sugary tea or coffee
- Eat junk foods
- Overeat
- Eat between meals
- Eat at night
- Drink excessively

BREAKFAST

IN

Continue with the phase one breakfast options. One non

fattening meal under your belt bodes well for the rest of the day. After breakfast don't eat until lunchtime.

OUT

Craving for carbohydrate is at its peak first thing in the morning when your brain needs energy, so when breakfast out is on the cards a strong resolve is needed. A sticky bun and a sweetened designer coffee topped with whipped cream, or a fizzy drink and a cigarette are unwise options. Pick one of these instead:

- Egg, sausage, baked beans and brown toast
- Bacon and egg bap
- Fresh fruit salad and porridge
- Small pack of nuts and raisins, unsweetened natural yoghurt and a banana
- Cheese and salad sandwich and an apple
- Omelette, chips and tomato

Drinks – unsweetened tea, coffee, herb or fruit tea, milk or water

LUNCH

IN

Sandwich, salad or hot meal, it is up to you. Remember to restrict added sugar and fat. After lunch don't eat until dinner. See Table 17.1 for phase two suggested lunches.

110

Table 17.1
PHASE TWO SUGGESTED LUNCHES

Monday	black bean and quinoa salad★ grapefruit or cheese and tomato sandwich blueberries and natural yoghurt
Tuesday	beetroot, barley and cheese salad★ banana or chicken and avocado sandwich apple
Wednesday	mackerel and potato salad★ passion fruit and fromage frais or egg and cucumber sandwich pineapple
Thursday	mushroom omelette and new potatoes strawberries or prawn and salad sandwich fresh mango
Friday	chicken curry and rice (ready meal) kiwi fruit or hummus and olive sandwich pear

Saturday	homemade soup cheese and crispbread or four frankfurters, baked beans and cucumber orange
Sunday	baked fish goujons, green beans and mashed potato plum or roast beef, Brussels sprouts, Yorkshire pudding and roast potatoes flourless chocolate cake★★

★see salads (chapter 21)
★★ see desserts (chapter 22)

OUT

Having lunch out? Resist impulse purchases by planning ahead. Choose one of these and skip the soft drink, crisps and chocolate bar.

- Coffee shop prepared salad
- Soup and sandwich, wrap or traditional sushi (less than 10g fat per pack)
- Cold meat, bread, orange
- Salad bar (lower fat options), fruit salad

- Supermarket rotisserie chicken pieces, bread, tomato
- Chicken or lamb kebab in pita bread with salad (no oil)
- Cooked meal – meat/fish and potatoes/rice, vegetable or salad, fruit
- Packed lunch – homemade salads (see chapter 21) or a portion of cheese, meat, fish, nuts or hummus with bread or crispbread, and fruit and natural yoghurt

DINNER

IN

Have a ready meal for lunch; cook a homemade meal for dinner. Search online for low fat versions of your favourite dishes. Stick to a maximum of one dinner plate of food per main course. Think smaller portions if you hope to keep your weight stable. Include a low fat, low sugar homemade dessert if you like something sweet to finish your meal. See Table 17.2 for phase two suggested dinners.

| **Table 17.2** | |
PHASE TWO SUGGESTED DINNERS	
Monday	low fat chicken and butternut squash risotto baked apple★★ or vegetarian lasagne (ready meal) and green salad (no oil) apple
Tuesday	homemade soup ham omelette and sauté potatoes or mixed bean salad★ cheese and crispbread
Wednesday	pork chop and cauliflower cheese almond pudding★★ or fish and chips, peas apple sprinkle★★
Thursday	salmon and peanut salad★ stewed cherries★★ or homemade soup sausages, bubble and squeak and baked beans

Friday	meatballs, millet and spring greens
	stewed plums★★
	or
	baked fish, sweetcorn and carrots
	noodle pudding★★
Saturday	two fried eggs, oven chips, tomato and lettuce
	or
	chicken and mushroom casserole and rice
	apple charlotte★★
Sunday	tomato and avocado with lemon juice
	pasta salad★
	or
	Quorn cutlet and broccoli
	bread and butter pudding★★

★ see salads (chapter 21)
★★ see desserts (chapter 22)

Drinks – unsweetened tea, coffee, herb or fruit tea, water with fresh lemon or lime juice

OUT

Dine out too frequently and weight maintenance becomes no more than wishful thinking. Faced with tempting choices and excessive portions, it is easy to overeat. Think protein, minimise added sugar and fat and steer clear of higher energy desserts like stodgy puddings or pastries. If you must devour the bread basket, skip the potatoes; it's one or the other, definitely not both. As for those little bowls of olive oil and after dinner chocolates, give them a miss. Avoid sugary cocktails, limit beer to one pint and wine to one or two glasses. Special occasion? Let your hair down with desserts such as fruit sorbet, mousse, jelly or poached fruit – just don't add cream. See Table 17.3 for phase two eating out.

Table 17.3
PHASE TWO EATING OUT

Starters	Mains
smoked fish	grilled fish
traditional sushi	seafood
avocado and tomato	kebab
prawns	pork chop
grilled calamari	roast chicken
scallops	roast beef
melon and ham	lamb stew
mussels	venison
vegetable soup	steak
fish soup	sausages
chicken wings	hamburger
satay sticks	omelette
steamed dumplings	pasta with tomato
tandoori chicken	pasta with seafood
lamb tikka	vegetable ravioli
asparagus	Indian dal
mixed salad	
Greek salad	

Sides	Dessert
new potatoes	sorbet
mashed potatoes	ice cream
roast potatoes	fruit salad
jacket potato	berries
chips (small portion)	jelly
pasta	mousse
bread	summer pudding
couscous	poached fruit
steamed rice	
sweetcorn	
quinoa	
pulses	
vegetables	
salad	

18

FAQ

I am fed up with being overweight but I know that dieting does not work. What is different about CAN I HAVE CHIPS?

The diet in CAN I HAVE CHIPS? is a long term diet not a faddy diet. Go on a faddy diet and lose weight, but once you inevitably stop, the weight goes back on again and you end up a little fatter than before you started dieting. Then you go on another diet, lose again, stop, and you end up even fatter. This is how crash dieters gain more and more weight over time. It is not your fault; your body thinks it is starving so it switches on all the mechanisms it has to store food.

The only diets that have been proven effective for long term weight loss focus on higher amounts of protein and vegetables and limit carbohydrates to those that are harder to digest. They work because they create an energy deficit, without the hunger and food cravings common to faddy diets.

I am only a few pounds overweight. Will the diet still work?

Dieting gets more difficult as you approach normal body weight. Lose those pesky last few pounds by preparing all your meals from scratch. No matter how sincere your intentions, it is much harder to reach your ideal weight if you eat out.

Why may I eat bread but not pastry?

Although both bread and pastry are made from flour, pastry unlike bread contains large amounts of fat, sometimes sugar and no water, making it an energy dense food. When buying packaged bread, check the ingredients as speciality breads may include substantial amounts of added fat. Better still, make it yourself.

Can I mix and match during phase one?

As long as you eat no more than one serving of starchy food and one serving of protein per meal, you can mix and match and it won't affect your weight loss. At breakfast have one slice of bread and half a small can of beans instead of two slices of bread, or one egg and one sausage instead of two eggs. However, it is better to pick just one starchy food and one protein food per meal, because we tend to want to eat more in the presence of variety.

Why is pizza more fattening than meat and potatoes? They both contain protein and starchy carbohydrate.

Although pizza is nutritious because it contains cheese and tomato, it is energy dense and very tasty, therein lays the dilemma. One or two slices are never enough to satisfy your appetite and most pizzas exceed your energy requirements for one meal, particularly when you are trying to lose weight. Meat and potatoes are not only less fattening, they are also more satisfying so you don't want to eat as much.

Why is it important to include vegetables and fruit in the diet?

Eating plenty of vegetables helps you lose weight because they are bulky and fill you up yet supply very little energy. Include some at lunch and dinner. Lightly cook them and they are even less fattening.

Once you give up sugary drinks, desserts, biscuits and confectionary, you welcome the sweetness that fruit provides. In time, sugary foods will taste too sweet for your palate.

What is worse? Added sugar or added fat?

Both added sugar and added fat predispose to overeating. Fat makes food more palatable, whereas sugar interferes with appetite regulation and leads to food cravings. Although sugar is lower in energy than fat, sugar consumption is linked to long term health problems, therefore giving up sugar should be your priority. An added bonus is that by avoiding sugary foods your fat intake naturally falls as well.

How much resistant starch should I consume in order to obtain maximum benefit?

It is early days in resistant starch research. You won't see it on a list of food ingredients, so it is not possible to know exactly how much you are consuming. It is clear that you do not need excessive amounts to have a beneficial effect on fat burning and appetite suppression. Rich sources are partly milled grains and seeds, pulses, firm bananas and cold, cooked potatoes and pasta. Choose these foods in preference to pastries, cakes and biscuits.

I frequently eat supermarket sandwiches at lunchtime. Will my sandwich habit stop me losing weight?

Readymade sandwiches usually contain plenty of fatty mayonnaise and not much appetite suppressing protein. If you eat a store bought sandwich every day you may find it hard to lose any weight. Make them more acceptable by buying protein rich sandwiches low in added fat – less than 10g fat per pack. Better still; prepare them yourself with decent bread.

Potatoes have a high glycaemic index (GI), why are they permitted?

Potatoes are fat free, watery, and unlike sugar do not contain empty calories. They give the highest satisfaction per calorie of any food, and feeling fuller on less food is what you are seeking to achieve. Many communities eat them as the basis of their diets without suffering from obesity, so it is clear that potatoes don't make you fat. In fact studies show that there is no difference in weight loss between high and low GI diets containing the same amount of carbohydrate. Rather than worrying about GI values, it makes more sense to cut out soft drinks, sugary tea and coffee, and fatty snacks which stimulate your appetite.

Is it true that carbohydrates make you fat?

No single food makes you fat, only overeating does this. But fat rich refined carbohydrates like pastry, cakes and biscuits are more fattening than fat free, harder to digest carbohydrates like wholegrains and pasta.

I am following the suggested meal plan but my weight is not shifting.

Start by writing down everything that passes your lips. Check that you really are complying with the diet and not snacking, eating junk foods or adding sugar or fat to cooking.

Increase the amount of protein you eat at each meal and reduce your starchy food intake to half a standard mug. Go teetotal as your body burns alcohol before the other macronutrients, and up your activity levels by walking more. Although diet is far more important than exercise in helping you lose weight, it still makes a significant contribution.

Visit your GP and ask for a blood test to check out your thyroid gland, as problems with your thyroid may affect your metabolism.

I have a sweet tooth and find it difficult not to eat sugary foods.

Sugary foods such as confectionary, cakes and biscuits are fattening because they are energy dense and highly palatable. Giving them up is easier if you replace them with naturally sweet fruit. Whole fruits are hard to overeat because they contain fibre, but avoid juice as it is easy to drink the juice of several fruits at one sitting.

I live in a hostel without cooking facilities.

Following the diet without access to cooking facilities is difficult but it need not be impossible. For breakfast eat a couple of slices of heavy bread or four slices of wholegrain crispbread with cheese or nut butter. At lunchtime buy a protein rich hot meal. Many larger supermarkets and most high streets have a cafe. Eat a piece of fresh fruit or nuts and raisins instead of a sugary dessert and avoid soft drinks. For your evening meal, choose from sliced cold meats, cooked chicken, tuna or sardines. Add some prepared carrot sticks or a tomato, and some pulses, sweetcorn or a banana. Finish your meal with natural yoghurt and a piece of fruit.

I need to lose 10 stone, how many pounds can I hope to lose a week?

Expect to lose one stone in the first month if you follow the diet carefully. After that be pleased with two pounds a week for the next month and one pound a week till you reach a healthy weight. Remember that as your weight drops, so must your food intake. Slim people need less food than their heavier friends.

Expect two steps forward and one step back. As long as you don't cave in to the lure of fast foods and sugary drinks, you can look forward to reaching your goal without becoming a diet bore. By this time you will be used to eating a satisfying meal three times a day without recourse to snacks.

Why are diet drinks not permitted?

On the face of it, diet drinks are the answer to your prayers as artificial sweeteners contain virtually no calories and are at least two hundred times sweeter than sucrose (table sugar). However, by getting used to so much sweetness, the normal sweet flavours of fruit and other sweet foods such as grains seem bland by comparison, making you less likely to consume them, and you continue to crave concentrated sugars.

Can I take things slowly as I don't think I can change everything at once?

Going cold turkey is appealing as it promises quick weight loss. But taking one step at a time is an equally valid approach, allowing you to prepare yourself for the way you are going to eat for the rest of your life. Start by eating three meals a day of real food containing minimal added sugar and fat. Then give up all soft drinks including fruit juice, and sugary tea and coffee. The final step is to stop eating between meals. You are now ready to follow the daily menus.

On holidays I let myself go and come back several pounds heavier.

However bad you've been, don't be tempted to use popular crash diets as they lead to rebound weight gain. This diet is designed to help you develop good eating habits, but you need to be consistent. On your return, carry on where you left off and the excess pounds will soon disappear. When you next take a break you will be less inclined to abandon the diet completely. In time your new way of eating becomes so ingrained that maintaining your weight when away from home becomes (almost) second nature.

I have a busy social life and often eat too much. What should I do?

Food binges lead to obesity, but practise the skills needed to put you in charge of what goes into your mouth and soon your lack of self control is but a distant memory.

I don't follow the rules every day, should I give up?

Losing weight? Then you are beginning to take on board the concepts of the diet. Over time good days exceed the bad, your weight falls further, and before long you will be reluctant to return to your old fattening eating habits.

My weight is dropping but the change of diet is giving me indigestion.

A sudden increase in your intake of fibre and resistant starch may cause flatulence or heartburn. Temporarily cut back on pulses, wholegrains, bananas and pasta, and obtain your starches from bread, and starchy vegetables such as parsnips and freshly cooked potatoes. Try to work out which foods are the culprits.

Consuming fruit at the same time as other foods sometimes results in discomfort. Eat fruit on an empty stomach, either one hour before your meal or three hours after a meal. It won't affect your rate of weight loss, but resist temptation to substitute a fatty snack for fruit.

19

THE BOTTOM LINE

- Fruit is not fattening
- Vegetables are not fattening
- Potatoes are not fattening
- Rice is not fattening
- Wholegrains are not fattening
- Heavy bread is not fattening
- Pasta is not fattening
- Eggs are not fattening
- Meat is not fattening
- Fish is not fattening
- Milk is not fattening
- Cheese is not fattening
- Natural unsweetened yoghurt is not fattening
- Pulses are not fattening
- Nuts are not fattening
- Seeds are not fattening
- Alcohol consumption in moderation is not fattening

- Added sugar is fattening
- Added oils and fats are fattening
- Soft drinks are fattening

- Sweet tea and coffee are fattening
- Fruit juices are fattening
- Chocolate is fattening
- Sweets are fattening
- Pastries are fattening
- Cakes are fattening
- Biscuits are fattening
- Eating between meals is fattening
- Skipping meals is fattening
- Night eating is fattening
- Large portions are fattening
- Fast foods are fattening
- Junk foods are fattening

So now you know how to lose weight and keep it off without hunger or food cravings. Take one meal at a time, and if you fall off the wagon don't wait until the next day, get back on it straightaway. A few slip-ups won't matter, it's remembering the principles, that is important – three meals a day of real food low in added sugar and fat, no sugary drinks and no snacking between meals.

Enjoy what you are planning to have for your supper and yes, you can have chips.

Bon Appétit

Louise

20

SERVING SUGGESTIONS

Experienced cooks look away now, no need to get upset being told the obvious. Mastered the art of tea making? Combining basic foods and applying heat to them is no more complicated. Scoff pie and chips at the pub washed down by a few pints and stay fat, or spend some of your precious time in the kitchen and slim down. Of course it is possible not to cook and lose weight but it is much more challenging and invariably more expensive.

Learn the basics and watch the pounds dissolve. But how, when you go to work, feed the kids, clean the flat, walk the dog, do the ironing and only have a microwave? Invest in a mini oven with hob; it will soon pay for itself. Save time by cooking enough food for two days, cooling it quickly before refrigerating at 4°C. Meat, fish, tofu, Quorn, eggs or pulses combined with grains, pasta or potatoes and served with a green salad or a vegetable, make a quick and easy meal. Just follow the golden rule – make sure that the amount of cooked starchy food does not exceed what you can fit in a standard mug (250ml).

Grains

Wholegrains – rice, quinoa, millet or barley – are less fattening than flour as they are harder for your body to process. They do not require the addition of fat to make them palatable. Allow about 50g of raw grain per serving and rinse before preparation. They cook quicker if presoaked for half an hour in enough water to cover them by 1cm.

To cook rice, quinoa or millet, bring them to the boil in the soaking water, turn off the heat after one minute, cover with a close fitting lid and leave to steam until cooked – about twenty minutes. Simmer barley until it is soft but still has bite. Basmati rice is the least fattening rice.

Pasta

Cook pasta by adding it to lightly salted boiling water. Use one portion fresh pasta or 65g dried pasta per person. Take pasta off the heat when it is still a little chewy *(al dente)*, drain and add the heated sauce. A mug of cooked pasta with meat balls, seafood, lentils or bolognaise sauce makes a filling supper. Serve with a mixed salad (no oil).

Pulses

A good source of vegetable protein, eat one portion of pulses (beans) a day to boost your metabolism.

5 servings

200g dried pulses
1 dessertspoon oil or butter

1 onion
2 cloves garlic
Fresh or dried ginger
Seasoning

Rinse 200g dried pulses, discard any stones and cover with plenty of water. Soak larger pulses overnight, smaller lentils and split peas only need thirty minutes. Drain and rinse the pulses. Cover with fresh water, boil with the lid off for five minutes to reduce the flatulent effect and skim off any white froth that forms.

Soften finely chopped onion, crushed garlic and minced ginger in the oil over a low heat. Add the pulses and cooking water. Simmer until cooked but not falling apart, adding more water as necessary. Towards the end of cooking time, season with salt, pepper or a little dried vegetable bouillon.

Potatoes

Serve potatoes with meat, fish, eggs, cheese, pulses, tofu or Quorn. Cooked, cooled and reheated potatoes contain significant resistant starch, so keep some handy in the fridge at 4°C for up to forty-eight hours.

Boiled Potatoes

Peel old potatoes, cut into similar sized pieces and boil in lightly salted water for about twenty minutes until soft all the way through. New potatoes do not need peeling before boiling. They cook quicker than old potatoes.

Steamed Potatoes

Steam new potatoes in a steamer, or place them in a sieve over simmering water for twenty minutes until soft.

Sautéed Potatoes

Sautéing is a tasty way to reheat boiled or steamed potatoes. Cut cold potatoes into slices and sauté with some diced onion in a non stick pan sprayed with oil. Cook until browned on both sides. Season and serve with omelette or sausages.

Baked Potatoes

Wash the potatoes but do not peel them. Prick and bake in a hot oven until soft (about one hour). Add grated cheese and beans. Microwave to reheat left over baked potatoes.

Roast Potatoes

Peel roasting potatoes and simmer for ten minutes in unsalted water. Drain and allow the steam to escape. Heat a little oil in a roasting pan. Add potatoes and salt lightly. Roast on the top shelf of a hot oven for one hour, turning occasionally, until browned and cooked through. Reheat leftover roast potatoes in the oven.

Mashed Potatoes

Peel potatoes and simmer until soft. Drain and allow the steam to escape. Mash with a little milk, salt and pepper.

Bubble and Squeak

Mix left over mashed potato with leftover cooked cabbage (or other vegetable) and sauté in a non stick frying pan sprayed with oil. Serve with eggs or meat.

Potato Salad

Shop bought potato salad often contains more mayonnaise than potato. Make your own, much less fattening, and it tastes better. Serve with cold meats or salmon.

2 medium potatoes per person
1 teaspoon mayonnaise or olive oil per person
Lemon juice
A few raisins
Spring onion, chives or parsley

Boil or steam new potatoes. Let them cool for thirty minutes before removing the skins (optional) and cutting into chunks. Add mayonnaise or olive oil, lemon juice, raisins, and sliced spring onions, chives or chopped parsley. Mix carefully by hand so the potatoes do not break up, season with salt and black pepper.

Meat

Cook meat straight from the fridge and it may end up tough, so remove it from the fridge a couple of hours before cooking to allow the fibres to relax. Steak is expensive but it is tender, it cooks quickly and there is no waste. Allow between 100g – 150g per person. Brush or wipe the steak with a little oil and do not grease the pan. Sear in a hot pan, then turn down the heat and cook for about three minutes on each side depending on how well you like your steak cooked. Leave it to rest on a warm plate before serving with chips or rice, and some mixed green leaves and grated carrot (no oil).

To roast a joint of meat or a chicken, season it with salt and pepper and a few herbs, rub it with a little balsamic vinegar and place it on a baking tray in a medium oven (for timings see pack label or ask butcher). Braising is the best way to cook a cheaper, and usually tougher, cut of meat. Place it in a closed casserole with some root vegetables and a small glass of wine. Cook in a medium oven for forty-five minutes, and then a low oven until tender – about two hours.

Cool leftovers thoroughly before refrigerating at 4°C. Reheat slices of meat or chicken by sautéing with a chopped onion or pepper and some sliced mushrooms. Add some black bean or tomato sauce, chutney or pesto. Serve with grains, pasta, potatoes, sweetcorn or pulses, and salad (no oil).

Fish

Fish cooks quicker than most meats, but it must be either very fresh or frozen and cooked on a low heat as it doesn't take kindly to being overcooked. Place 100g – 150g per person of fish fillets in the centre of a large piece of lightly greased foil. Cover with a few slices of tomato or some sliced olives, and add a squeeze of lemon or a splash of white wine. Make a loose parcel with the foil and bake in a medium oven for about fifteen minutes (fresh fish) or until the fish flakes easily.

Cook fish on the hob by gently frying fillets in a little oil or butter with some chilli pepper, balsamic vinegar or chopped parsley. Feeling virtuous? Try grilling your fish and dowsing it in lemon juice.

Eggs

Eggs are easy to cook and very nutritious. Keep some handy for quick and filling meals, particularly breakfast. Use them by their best-before date.

Boiled Egg

Fill a small pan with water. Carefully place the egg into boiling water so that it is completely covered. Boil for four and half minutes for soft boiled, and ten minutes for hard boiled.

Fried Egg

Spray a non stick frying pan with oil. Heat the pan, crack the egg and slide it into the pan. Turn down the heat and cook for a few minutes. Flip the egg over (optional) and cook for a further ten seconds, season with salt and pepper and serve on toast.

Scrambled Egg

Beat two eggs with a fork. Add the eggs to a pan greased with butter, and stir with a wooden spoon over a very low heat until just cooked, season with salt and pepper.

Porridge

2 servings

Oatmeal makes the best porridge. It takes longer to cook than rolled oats but is well worth the wait. Put one cup of coarse oatmeal into a medium pan with two cups of water and one cup of milk. Bring to the boil stirring constantly. Add a pinch of salt and simmer gently for five minutes. Turn off the heat and leave it to stand with a tight fitting lid until cooked (about twenty minutes). It can be made the night before and reheated in the microwave. Serve with one teaspoon maple syrup per person and some flaked almonds.

If you are short of time, add water and some milk to rolled porridge oats and cook for a few minutes.

Cooked Breakfast

1 serving

Heat a non stick pan sprayed with oil. Fry a good quality sausage on a moderate heat and discard the fat that is released. Add one rasher of bacon, half a large tomato and some sliced mushrooms. When the sausage, bacon, tomato and mushrooms are cooked, place them on a warmed plate. Fry an egg then wipe the pan clean and heat some baked beans, or prepare a piece of toast made from heavy bread.

Fruit Salad

6 servings

Cut up one banana, two satsumas or one orange, twenty grapes, a large apple and two kiwi fruit. Add the juice of half a lemon to stop the fruit browning. Refrigerate and serve with one dessertspoon natural yoghurt, fromage frais or ricotta cheese. Do not add sugar.

Pasta Combos

Plain boiled pasta is a tasteless affair. Add one of these combos to freshly cooked pasta and make your meal both filling and slimming. Flavour with black bean or tomato based sauce, balsamic vinegar or pesto. Serve hot or cold. During phase one, limit cooked pasta to one standard mug (250ml) per meal. When you reach maintenance your main course should not exceed what you can easily fit on one dinner plate.

- black beans and diced feta cheese
- sweetcorn and crushed hazelnuts
- shredded canned tuna or salmon and flaked almonds
- diced cooked chicken breast and sliced spring onion
- sundried tomatoes and sliced cooked vegetarian or meat sausage
- grated cheese and edamame beans
- sliced artichoke hearts and black olives

Salad Combos

Lettuce, tomato and cucumber is not the only salad. Try these easy to prepare, protein rich salad combos. Season with balsamic vinegar or lemon juice and serve with a baked potato or a few new potatoes for a satisfying summer lunch.

- smoked salmon, cucumber and watercress
- tomato, avocado and mozzarella

- chick peas, grated courgette, tomato and olives
- chicory, cheddar cheese and tomato
- tuna, sweetcorn and red pepper
- hardboiled egg, rocket and goats cheese
- pear, blue cheese, and green leaves
- salami, white beans and apple
- beetroot, orange and walnut

Sandwich Combos

Forget bog standard sandwiches heavy in fat and light on protein. Open sandwiches made with good bread, preferably sourdough, are infinitely preferable and a lot tastier. Cut two medium slices of bread and spread both of them with a little mayonnaise, butter or mustard and one of these sandwich combos. Serve with a few green leaves.

- liver paté and chicory
- swiss cheese, tomato and parsley
- brie and grapes
- mashed hardboiled egg and olives
- ham and chutney
- chicken and avocado
- hummus (1 dessertspoon) and rocket
- smoked salmon, yoghurt and cucumber
- ricotta cheese and radish
- prawn and salad
- pastrami and pickled cucumber
- goats cheese and spring onion

Grain Combos

Rice is not the only grain. Ring the changes with nutty tasting quinoa, hearty barley or warming millet. Add one of these hot cooked combos to freshly cooked grain. Stir through a dollop of black bean, spicy mango, tomato or any other low fat sauce. During phase one limit cooked grains to one standard mug (250ml) per meal.

- stir fried beef, chicken or pork, and broccoli florets
- butter beans and leeks
- red kidney beans and mushrooms
- leftover roast lamb and onions
- white fish and peas
- tofu and red pepper
- smoked haddock, hardboiled egg and parsley
- sausage and broad beans

21

SIMPLE SOUPS AND SALADS

With virtually no cooking skills you can succeed at losing weight. But plan to keep it off and learning how to prepare simple dishes becomes a necessity. With thousands of recipes online, in newspapers and in cookery books, there can be no shortage of inspiration. Most are off the radar, but a few are rich in real food – wholegrains, fruit, vegetables, pulses, and proteins – and low in added sugar and fat.

Yes, cooking can be arduous and you may have little inclination to waste your precious free time in the kitchen rustling up delicious meals. There is no easy answer to this dilemma. Employ a chef, find a wife or a domesticated husband who is turned off by your wobbly bits, or cut down on watching TV, gaming, or painting your nails.

Master a repertoire of hearty winter soups and interesting summer salads, and maintaining your weight loss becomes a real possibility because soups and salads are naturally low in energy. Making soup from scratch takes effort, so prepare enough to last a few days, or freeze it in portions. During the colder months, a lunch of soup, heavy bread, cheese or meat and a piece of fruit, keeps you going until dinner time without the urge to snack. In summer, salads rich in protein and grains leave you feeling satisfied but not lethargic.

Soups

Most soups are made from a base of two or three vegetables. Sweating helps soften them and draws out the flavours. The idea isn't to brown or caramelise them – instead the mellow aromas from the vegetables should mingle with the rest of the dish without dominating it.

For a standard soup base, chop one large onion, two sticks of celery and a couple of carrots. Heat one dessertspoon of olive oil in a large pan and add the soup base vegetables, the vegetables from your chosen recipe and a pinch of salt. With the lid firmly closed, adjust the heat so you hear a gentle sizzle and sweat for about ten minutes stirring occasionally.

At the end of the sweating time, improve the flavour of your soup by adding a glug of sherry or half glass of white wine, allowing it to evaporate before incorporating the remaining ingredients. These recipes contain dried vegetable bouillon to save time, but homemade vegetable or chicken stock gives a superior flavour.

Blending the cooked soup is easy using an electric blender, but you can mash it with a potato masher or push it through a sieve. Dilute with water or milk if the finished soup is too thick for your taste.

Butternut Squash, Lentil and Ginger Soup

6 servings

Soup base
50g small dried lentils
1 medium butternut squash
1 litre water
2cm piece of fresh ginger or a ½ tsp dried ginger
Fresh or dried red chilli pepper
2 level tsp vegetable bouillon

Rinse the lentils and soak for thirty minutes. Peel the squash, discard the seeds and cut into chunks. Mix the squash with the soup base vegetables and sweat. Add the water, the lentils, the ginger and a little fresh or dried chilli pepper. Boil for five minutes, skimming off any white froth that forms and simmer until cooked, adding the vegetable bouillon near the end of the cooking time. Blend the cooled soup and season to taste.

Brussels Sprouts and Chestnut Soup

6 servings

Soup base
250g fresh Brussels sprouts
1 litre of water
1 small can or vacuum pack of peeled chestnuts
2 level tsp vegetable bouillon
½ tsp ground cumin seed
Parsley
Natural yoghurt

Remove any damaged leaves from the sprouts. Add the

sprouts to the soup base vegetables and sweat. Add the water, chestnuts, vegetable bouillon and ground cumin and simmer for thirty minutes. Blend the cooled soup, season and serve decorated with chopped parsley and a teaspoon of yoghurt.

Leek, Parsnip and Garlic Soup

6 servings

Soup base
4 leeks
2 parsnips
4 cloves garlic
1 litre water
2 level tsp vegetable bouillon
Parmesan

Slice the leeks and cut the peeled parsnips into chunks. Combine with the soup base vegetables and sweat. Add the crushed garlic cloves, water and bouillon. Simmer until the vegetables are soft. Blend the cooled soup, season and serve with grated parmesan.

Cauliflower, Blue Cheese and Nutmeg Soup

6 servings

Soup base
1 medium cauliflower
1 large potato
1 litre water
2 level tsp vegetable bouillon
50g blue cheese

Nutmeg
Fresh coriander

Divide the cauliflower into florets discarding the tough part of the stalk. Cut the peeled potato into chunks. Combine the cauliflower and potato with the soup base vegetables and sweat. Add the water and the bouillon. Simmer until the vegetables are tender. Crumble the cheese into the soup and grate in some nutmeg. Allow the cheese to melt. Blend the cooled soup, season and decorate with coriander leaves.

Chicken, Mushroom and Barley Soup

6 servings

5 whole dried mushrooms or 2 tablespoons sliced dried mushrooms
2 tablespoons barley
2 chicken leg quarters or 6 wings
1 litre water
4 large carrots
1 level tsp vegetable bouillon
Fresh parsley

Rinse the mushrooms and cover with water. Rinse the barley and leave to soak. Place the chicken and water in a saucepan and bring to the boil, carefully removing the scum that forms. Add the sliced carrots and the mushrooms with the soaking water to the pan. Simmer for thirty minutes then add the drained barley and the parsley including the stalks. Simmer for a further thirty minutes. Taste; add the bouillon if required and some more water if too much has evaporated. Remove the chicken and shred a little, adding it to the soup. Season and serve. Any leftover chicken can be mixed with a little mayonnaise and curry powder and eaten cold.

Pea, Watercress and Lemon Grass Soup

6 servings

Soup base
500g frozen peas
Bunch water cress
6 fresh mint leaves or 1 tsp dried mint
Stick lemon grass
1 litre water
2 level tsp vegetable bouillon
Natural yoghurt

Sweat the soup base vegetables. Add the peas, chopped watercress, fresh or dried mint, a crushed stick of lemon grass, water and the vegetable bouillon and simmer for thirty minutes. Remove the lemon grass, blend the cooled soup and season. Serve hot or cold, decorated with a teaspoon of natural yoghurt.

Jerusalem Artichoke and Carrot Soup

6 servings

Soup base
500g carrots
300g Jerusalem artichokes
1 litre water
2 level tsp vegetable bouillon
Pinch cayenne pepper

Add the chopped peeled carrots and artichokes to the soup

base vegetables and sweat. Add the water and the bouillon and simmer for about forty-five minutes or until the vegetables are soft. Blend the cooled soup and season to taste with cayenne pepper. Dilute if too thick.

Red Lentil and Sun Dried Tomato Soup

6 servings

Soup base
200g dried red lentils
1 tablespoon sundried tomatoes
½ tsp ground cumin seed
½ tsp cinnamon
1 litre water
2 level tsp vegetable bouillon
1 small green pepper

Soak the lentils for at least thirty minutes, drain and rinse. Sweat the soup base vegetables, then add the chopped tomatoes, lentils, cumin, cinnamon and water. Boil for five minutes, skim off any white froth that forms, then simmer for one hour. Add the bouillon towards the end of the cooking time. Blend the cooled soup, season and serve decorated with finely diced green pepper.

Summer Salads

These summer salads rich in protein and low in added fat are easy to prepare. They serve four people as a main course and may be safely stored in the fridge at 4°C for two days.

Pasta Salad

4 servings

260g dried pasta
12 cherry or 6 medium tomatoes
16 stoned olives
50g nuts
2 tsp balsamic vinegar
50g parmesan shavings or grated parmesan
Fresh coriander, parsley or watercress

While the pasta is cooking, chop the tomatoes, slice the olives and lightly crush the nuts. Drain the pasta while it is still slightly chewy. Stir through the balsamic vinegar and then add the cheese, tomatoes, olives and nuts. Pour the salad into large flat serving dish. Combine with the herbs or watercress just before serving.

Salmon and Peanut Salad

4 servings

200g basmati rice
213g can salmon
4 dessertspoons lemon juice
50g unsalted peanuts (or other nuts)
4 spring onions
Half cucumber
Black pepper

While the rice is cooking, lightly shred the drained salmon and combine with the lemon juice, peanuts and sliced spring onion. Add them to the warm freshly cooked rice and season with black pepper. Stir through peeled and diced cucumber just before serving.

Beetroot, Barley and Cheese Salad

4 servings

200g barley
3 medium cooked beetroot (250g)
Juice of one large orange
200g Edam cheese
1 small can sweetcorn
Fresh parsley
Black pepper

While the barley is cooking, dice the beetroot and mix with the orange juice. Cube the cheese and combine with the drained sweetcorn and freshly cooked barley. Pour into a shallow dish and scatter the beetroot on top. Sprinkle with ample amounts of chopped parsley and season with black pepper.

Mixed Bean Salad

4 servings

1 large can (400g) mixed beans
2 large eating apples
200g Feta cheese
2 dessertspoons lemon/lime juice
Black pepper
Mixed leaves

Drain and rinse the beans. Core the apples, cut them into

small chunks and put in a bowl with cold water and lemon juice to prevent browning. Combine the beans, drained apples, crumbled feta and two dessertspoons lemon or lime juice. Season the salad with black pepper and stir through the leaves just before serving.

Mackerel and Potato Salad

4 servings

8 medium salad potatoes
4 smoked mackerel fillets (about 280g)
I large red pepper
1 level dessertspoon horseradish sauce
1 medium lemon
Black pepper
Bunch watercress

Boil or steam the potatoes and leave to cool. Skin and shred the mackerel fillets, dice the red pepper and cut the potatoes into chunks. Combine them with the horseradish sauce and the juice from the lemon. Season with freshly ground black pepper and add the roughly chopped watercress just before serving.

Black Bean and Quinoa Salad

4 servings

200g quinoa
4 medium tomatoes (or 1 red pepper)
12 radishes
4 spring onions
400g can/carton black beans

2 tablespoons lemon juice
Salt and pepper
Chives/parsley/coriander

While the quinoa is cooking, slice the tomatoes, the radishes, and the white parts of the spring onions. Combine with the drained and rinsed black beans and lemon juice. Stir through the warm freshly cooked quinoa and season to taste. Put the salad into a shallow serving dish. Sprinkle over a generous amount of chopped chives, parsley or coriander just before serving.

22

LESS FATTENING DESSERTS

Love desserts? Feel free to indulge in one of these low added sugar and low added fat desserts, but only once you reach maintenance and are not actively trying to lose weight. They may look calorific, but are relatively innocuous compared to shop bought offerings with their generous portion size and high energy density.

Limit yourself to one serving of dessert a day and no seconds either. Use a teaspoon and make it last longer. Don't ruin your efforts by adding cream or ice cream as you may as well eat a store bought chocolate sponge or syrup pudding and save yourself the bother of cooking. Custard anyone?

Baked Apple

1 large cooking apple per person (or 2 eating apples)
Raisins
Cinnamon
1 tsp brown sugar per apple

Bramleys make the best baked apples. Core the apples and

slice horizontally through the skin all the way round. Place in a baking dish so that they fit snugly. Half fill the cavities with raisins and a sprinkle of cinnamon. Pour 1cm water into the bottom of the dish and stir in one teaspoon of sugar per apple. Cook in a medium oven for forty-five minutes or until soft all the way through. Serve hot or cold with a tablespoon of natural yoghurt.

Bread No Butter Pudding

6 servings

8 small slices wholemeal bread
20g raisins
2 large eggs
400ml semi skimmed milk
2 heaped tsp honey
Pinch nutmeg

Cut the bread slices in half diagonally, sprinkle the raisins between the slices and overlap them in a greased oven dish. Beat the eggs, milk, honey and nutmeg and pour over the bread. Leave the pudding to stand for twenty minutes to allow the bread to swell. Put the dish in a baking tin containing enough water to reach half way up the dish and cook until the custard is set, the bread is puffed up and the top is crisp – about forty-five minutes in a medium oven. Serve warm.

Stewed Cherries

4 servings

450g cherries
3 tsp brown sugar
Ginger

Remove the stalks and wash the cherries. Place them in a pan with the sugar, a sprinkle of ginger and a tablespoon of water. Stir and simmer gently for about twenty minutes. The fruit will release water during cooking. Remove the cherries carefully then simmer the sauce until it starts to become syrupy – about five minutes. Pour over the cherries. Eat warm or cold with a dollop of natural yoghurt.

Stewed Plums

6 servings

18 small ripe plums
3 tsp brown sugar
1 level tsp butter
½ vanilla pod
Flaked almonds

Put the washed plums, sugar and butter in a pan with a splash of water. Split the vanilla pod and scrape out seeds. Add the seeds and the empty pod to the pan. Simmer for ten minutes, or until the plums are cooked through but not falling apart. Pour into a shallow dish, carefully remove the stones and sprinkle some flaked almonds over the top.

Almond Pudding

10 servings

4 large eggs
120g caster sugar
120g ground almonds (or hazelnuts)

Beat the eggs and sugar until thick and pale. Add the ground almonds and combine well. Pour into a greased oven dish lined with baking paper and bake in a moderate oven for about thirty-five minutes until a skewer inserted into the pudding comes out clean. Remove the pudding from the dish and cool on a wire rack. Lightly dust with a little caster sugar. Serve with stewed cherries and a blob of natural yoghurt.

Noodle Pudding

8 servings

140g vermicelli noodles
1 large egg
100g pot unsweetened fruit compote
125g ricotta cheese
2 level dessertspoons brown sugar
1 tablespoon raisins
½ vanilla pod
Nutmeg

Cook the vermicelli *al dente,* it will continue to cook in the oven. Beat the egg and combine it with the fruit compote, ricotta and sugar, then add the raisins, the scraped out seeds from the vanilla pod and the noodles. Pour into a greased baking dish. Sprinkle the top with nutmeg. Bake in a

moderate over for one hour loosely covered with foil. Best
served warm with a few berries or orange segments.

Apple Charlotte

6 servings

850g cooking apples
2 level dessertspoons brown sugar
1 tsp cinnamon
1 unwaxed lemon
8 small slices wholegrain or wholemeal bread
butter

Peel, core and chop each apple into eight pieces. Simmer
them in a splash of water with half the sugar and the
cinnamon until just soft but retaining their shape (about ten
minutes). Add the grated rind and juice of the washed lemon.
Spread butter very thinly on both sides of the bread and cut
the slices in half diagonally. Line the sides of a medium oven
proof dish with ten of the sixteen pieces of bread so that they
overlap and the points face upwards. Fill the dish with the
stewed apple and cover with the remaining six pieces of bread.
Sprinkle with the rest of the sugar and bake in a moderate
oven for thirty to forty minutes until the top is browned and
crisp. Serve with natural yoghurt.

Apple Sprinkle

4 servings

40g mixed unsalted nuts
30g brown sugar
6 eating apples
1 tsp butter
1 tsp cinnamon

Lightly crush the nuts and mix with the sugar. Peel and core the apples and cut into chunks. Rinse the chunks and simmer them with the butter and cinnamon until softened but retaining their shape. Put the apple in a shallow oven proof dish, sprinkle the sweetened nuts and cook in a medium oven for about twenty minutes, taking care not to allow the nut mixture to burn.

Flourless Chocolate Cake

8 servings

3 large eggs
65g caster sugar
125g ricotta cheese
30g ground almonds
30g best quality cocoa powder

Preheat a medium oven. Beat the eggs with the sugar until creamy. Add the cheese and combine thoroughly, then fold in the almonds and cocoa powder. Pour into a small non stick loaf tin lined with baking parchment. Bake for thirty minutes. The centre should still be moist. Cool for five minutes then turn out on to a wire rack. Serve warm or cold with stewed apple, stewed cherries or a spoon of natural yoghurt.